THE
SIRT DIET

JACQUELINE WHITEHART

The new SUPERFOODS that will help you
LOSE WEIGHT FAST

COOKBOOK

HarperCollins*Publishers*
1 London Bridge Street,
London SE1 9GF

www.harpercollins.co.uk

3 5 7 9 10 8 6 4

Photography © Tom Regester
Food stylist: Becks Wilkinson
Prop stylist: Wei Tang

A catalogue record for this book is
available from the British Library.

PB ISBN: 978-0-00-816336-5
EB ISBN: 978-0-00-816337-2

Printed and bound in Great Britain by
Clays Ltd, St Ives plc.

MIX
Paper from
responsible sources
FSC™ C007454

CONTENTS

INTRODUCTION

Welcome to a new style of diet, which is first and foremost about eating more of the right foods and less of the wrong ones. *The SIRT Diet Cookbook* is chock-full of diet-friendly advice, planners, tips and fantastic recipes, with everything you need to start eating right today.

I'm just your average working mum, juggling child commitments and a haphazard career. Along the way I have experimented with many diets: some good (for a time); some disastrous from day one. I genuinely know how diets work because I've truly been there ... I feel like I've tried them all! I know how you start the day with good intentions, feeling virtuous with a low-calorie breakfast, but are hungry by lunch and ready to scream by teatime. Finally, you sit down at the end of the day with a drink in one hand and a cake in the other, wondering where it all went wrong.

I have ended up with a new outlook on dieting and the diet industry. If a diet is all about cutting back and restrictions, it's difficult to keep it up for long. One day your willpower just disappears, you crash and burn, and end up feeling like a failure. This diet is different; it's all about the superfoods. SIRT superfoods really do boost your metabolism, converting body fat to energy and breaking the cycle of feast and famine by naturally reducing your cravings for junk food.

I have had to believe in myself to come this far on my diet journey. After becoming known as a healthy-eating expert by way of the 5:2 Diet, I started to let my own standards slip as family life got in the way. This led to inevitable weight gain and a huge dip in my confidence. But I've never been afraid to start again and try new things. I am a self-experimenter by nature so when the opportunity came along to start the SIRT Diet, I couldn't wait. The results have been extraordinary. Not just weight-loss. My energy levels are up and my skin glows. I feel the best I've done in years.

The SIRT Diet is not just red wine and chocolate. It's also green tea, kale and lots of fruit and vegetables. It's so straightforward anyone and everyone should follow it. If you're ready to try something new and embrace the SIRT way of eating, you won't regret it.

Follow my simple and complete plan and lose weight, tone up and look great.

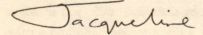

REAL FOOD, REAL RECIPES AND A DIET THAT REALLY WORKS

The SIRT Diet Cookbook teaches you to eat the right foods – natural and flavoursome foods as diverse as kale and chocolate – that all contain a newly discovered type of superfood, called SIRT foods.

SIRT foods are special because they are the key to unlocking significant genes in our bodies – the genes that regulate our metabolism and help us to resist disease.

The headlines are true: red wine and dark chocolate are both SIRT foods and can help you lose weight. But behind the headlines there is so much more to this diet and this is what *The SIRT Diet Cookbook* seeks to explain. Find out what SIRT foods really are, discover the best SIRT foods for you to eat, understand how these superfoods really boost your metabolism and control your food cravings. Best of all, this cookbook is full of simple and amazing recipes that all include these incredible superfoods. Learn how to boost your SIRT foods by adding a few unusual ingredients. Spice things up with turmeric or mellow out with chocolate – the choice is yours.

MY JOURNEY

Following three successful books and a popular recipe blog, I've been an advocate of the two-day fasting diet for years. But perhaps inevitably I've got bored of fasting and to be totally honest, I've found fasting to be harder with less impressive results. In fact my food cravings started to increase, I ate more on days when I wasn't fasting and I started to gain weight.

I first found out about SIRT foods while trying to find an easier way to get the results of calorie restriction. In a scientific research paper, I read that there were two ways to activate the insulin-sensitive hormone IGF-1 (the one triggered by 5:2 and fasting). The first was calorie restriction and the second was specific trigger foods. Intrigued, I started to try and find out more. There hasn't been much about the diet in the press except a few tantalising newspaper articles with headlines shouting 'Eat more chocolate, drink more red wine'. These headlines are an oversimplification of a fantastic truth:

Eat SIRT foods such as kale, turmeric
and dark chocolate and they will help you
lose weight naturally.

If it sounds too good to be true, it's really not. These super-foods start a chain reaction inside you that makes your metabolism work more efficiently and allows you to make more effective use of the calories you consume. This naturally curbs your appetite, boosts your energy levels and fights inflammation. There's a lot more about the science behind SIRT foods and their key role in your metabolism in the section 'What are SIRT foods and why are they special?'

TOP TEN SIRT FOODS

1 Green tea
2 Red grapes and red wine
3 Kale
4 Dark chocolate
5 Ground turmeric

6 Onions
7 Citrus fruits
8 Olives and olive oil
9 Pomegranate
10 Soy beans and tofu

Green tea is the top of all SIRT foods, containing a rich source of catechins, the most powerful sirtuin activator scientifically identified. For this reason, drinking at least two cups of tea a day is considered to be one of the fundamentals of the SIRT Diet. What if you've never tried green tea and don't like the sound of it? You are not alone. Luckily I was in the same boat as you only a short while ago and I've got the complete guide to learning to love green tea. Take a look at the 'Living the Diet' section to find out more.

Go on, drink your green tea, eat your chocolate and guzzle your red wine. Look at the amazing benefits they bring:

- Triggering your metabolism to break down more fat
- Natural reduction in appetite and hunger pangs
- Converting fat to muscle without increasing exercise

WHAT ARE SIRT FOODS AND WHY ARE THEY SPECIAL?

SIRT foods are super antioxidants that activate the sirtuin genes in our body, producing an increased fat-burning response. In a nutshell, eating more of these foods will boost your metabolism and help you lose weight faster.

THE SIRTUIN GENES

There are seven sirtuin genes in humans, imaginatively named SIRT1 to SIRT7. Geneticists have done several studies on the sirtuins and have had positive results relating to increased lifespan, metabolism and anti-ageing. Scientists are only just beginning to understand the function of individual genes and there is a lot still to be done, particularly related to how the genes work together.

SIRT1, SIRT3 and SIRT4 function predominantly on the metabolism, with SIRT4 specifically related to insulin sensitivity. SIRT2, SIRT6 and SIRT7 have more anti-ageing tasks related to cell and DNA repair. The individual genes do not work in isolation, but in combination, in ways that we do not yet fully understand. What is abundantly clear is that the sirtuin family of genes are extremely valuable within the body and activating these genes makes us healthier, promotes weight-loss and helps us age gracefully. So how do we go about making these genes work better?

It has recently been established that there are two main triggers for the sirtuin genes. One is calorie restriction and the other is SIRT activators. Foods that contain a rich source of SIRT activators are collectively called SIRT foods.

Perhaps you've tried calorie restriction, fasting or the 5:2 Diet? They definitely work and can produce dramatic results but you need a lot of willpower to stick to the diets over the long term. What if there is an alternative, where you substitute special foods for fasting or calorie restriction? Not only that, but these special foods are easy to come by and are tasty, flavoursome and wholesome.

With a SIRT-rich diet, your genes benefit in a very similar way to calorie restriction … without restricting calories.

SIRTUINS AND YOUR HEALTH

When you activate the SIRT proteins in your body, they act as 'housekeepers' doing all the hard work that other genes don't or can't do. Sirtuins are a family of age-related proteins. The main role of sirtuins is to selectively regulate the activity of key genes responsible for metabolism and cell defence:

1 *Increase fat metabolism, burning more calories from fat*
It has been shown that SIRT activation shifts metabolism away from using glucose as an energy source, favouring fat synthesis.

2 *Reduce insulin response*
The hormone Insulin-like Growth Factor 1 (IGF-1) is proven to decrease as SIRT genes are activated. IGF-1 is produced in the liver and is similar to insulin. Its purpose in the body is to make cells grow and produce new cells. When levels of IGF-1 decrease, our body produces few new cells and concentrates on repairing old ones. This state of 'repair' is very beneficial as it slows down the ageing process.

3 *Fight inflammation*
Through their powerful antioxidant effect, sirtuins reduce oxidative stress, which has positive repercussions for cardiovascular protection and heart health.

HOW DO SIRTUINS HELP YOU LOSE WEIGHT?

Triggering your SIRT genes sparks a change in your metabolism that breaks down more fat cells. The activated SIRTs increase the amount of a neurotransmitter called norepinephrine, which is used by the nervous system as a signal to fat cells, telling them to break down fat. The signal telling the fat cell to convert fat to energy is stronger, increasing fat burning.

Want to burn more fat?

Drink green tea. Green tea combines SIRT activators and a (small) dose of caffeine. The caffeine enhances the effect of the SIRTs, meaning more fat is broken down.

Natural appetite suppressant effect

When the body breaks down fat, the fat is converted into energy. This energy is used immediately by the body. This has a positive effect on how you feel, giving your energy levels a boost and decreasing hunger.

Converting fat to muscle

Combining SIRTs with exercise boosts the fat-burning effect even further. If you exercise the energy released from fat cells is available for strengthening muscles.

In practice this means that if you follow the SIRT diet and exercise several times a week you will not only lose weight, but you will look and feel leaner as some of the weight has been converted into muscle.

For absolute peak fat-burning performance when exercising, drink two cups of green tea (for the SIRTs *and* the caffeine) within one hour before or after exercise.

SIRT FOODS

SIRT foods contain one (or more) of a very specific subset of bioactives. Bioactives are in turn part of a larger group of health-giving compounds called antioxidants. There are in fact seven substances that make up the SIRT food family, each of which activates the SIRTUIN genes. As with vitamins and minerals, a daily mix of different types gives the most benefit.

RESVERATROL

Perhaps the best known of the SIRT food family, resveratrol is a scientifically proven activator of the SIRT1 gene.
Found in: red wine, red grapes, chocolate

BERBERINE

Berberine is a trigger of the (normally) exercise-induced AMPK hormone. AMPK complements the SIRT family and activates the sirtuin genes.
Found in: turmeric

CATECHINS

Catechins are highly potent antioxidants that are strong triggers for the SIRT gene. Combining catechins with caffeine in green tea boosts the metabolic effects of both the catechins and the caffeine.

Found in: green tea

QUERCETIN

A versatile bioactive that can be found in most fruit and vegetables. The greatest concentration of quercetin is in red onions and parsley.

Found in: onions, apples, parsley, pomegranate

OMEGA-3 FATTY ACIDS

Try and eat oily fish at least once a week to get these essential fats, which the body can't make itself.

Found in: salmon, trout, mackerel

KAEMPFEROL

The 'leafy greens' bioactive. But can also be found in tea, leeks and strawberries. Eat as much of it as you can.

Found in: kale, broccoli, spinach

HYDROXYTYROSOL

The only bioactive antioxidant that works throughout the whole body, including the central nervous system.
Found in: olives, olive oil

ISOFLAVONES

Bioactive found predominantly in soy and its derivatives. As well as antioxidant properties, isoflavones influence our reproductive hormones and can act as a preventative for menopausal symptoms.
Found in: soya beans and tofu

It is important to understand that all of these SIRT foods contain not just one but a range of activators, each having different effects. The science behind how all the activators work together is only just beginning to be understood. By eating a large variety of these foods and eating them consistently and often, we can optimise our sirtuin genes and get the best results.

WHY NOT JUST TAKE A SUPPLEMENT?

There are various studies taking place right now, testing some, but not all, of the SIRT bioactives. Studies with concentrated resveratrol are ongoing but have yet to show the desired health improvements. This indicates that there are many aspects of the interaction of these compounds with our bodies that are not yet fully understood. The best approach is to take a variety of SIRTs within as many different, natural foodstuffs as possible.

THE MEDITERRANEAN DIET

The Mediterranean diet has long been synonymous with longevity and health. Ever since it was discovered that people living in the Mediterranean region had low rates of chronic diseases such as cancer and heart disease, people have been trying to pinpoint the root of its success. Key foods in the Mediterranean diet such as olive oil, red wine and plenty of fruit and vegetables are also key foods in the SIRT diet. This is no coincidence. One of the reasons the Mediterranean diet is so successful is the prevalence of SIRT foods.

Why not take it one step further and look at other healthy national diets. One of the healthiest in the world is the Japanese diet. Here we think of oily fish, soy, seaweed and green tea. These are some of the most important SIRT foods.

Combine the Mediterranean and Japanese diets and we end up with perhaps the healthiest diet of all time: the SIRT Diet.

NATURAL, AFFORDABLE
AND BALANCED

Looking at a cross-section of SIRT foods we find plenty of foods that are already part of a healthy diet. Fruits and vegetables figure highly with onions, green leafy vegetables and red grapes being some of the most SIRT-rich foods available. Fats are covered in the form of olive oil, the most versatile, natural and healthy oil there is. Some carbohydrates and proteins are also SIRT-rich; think tofu and beans, which both have a great balance of carbs and protein, and oily fish, which contains protein and omega-3 oils. It is likely, however, that you will need to supplement SIRT foods with some good carbs like basmati rice, wholemeal bread, pasta and oats. Chicken and some red meat are also needed to add more protein to the diet.

Don't be afraid to add lean proteins and good carbs to make a balanced diet; just think natural and cook from scratch wherever possible. The simple and sensible recipes in this book will help you do just that.

THE SIRT 5 A DAY

Ever heard of '5 a day'? Of course you have. The 5 a day of fruit and vegetables is one of the cornerstones of the British diet. It is taught in school and referred to in practically every healthy eating guideline around. In fact, I bet you know some of its intricacies too. Do potatoes count as one of your 5 a day? No. What about fruit juice? Yes. But only as one of your 5 a day, even if you drink more than one glass. It's a fantastically clear and useful concept that teaches us all the value of eating fruit and veg and encourages us to eat more of them.

When we follow the SIRT diet we can build on and work with our awareness of 5 a day to make the 'SIRT 5 a day' to help you keep track of the SIRTS you eat and make sure you're getting enough. Sounds simple? It really is. Get to know your SIRT foods and the quantities you need to eat by following the SIRT 5-a-day guidelines and you will be a SIRT diet convert in no time.

Here is the only 'guideline' you need to follow for daily SIRT goodness:

Eat 5 or more portions of SIRT foods every day, consuming the greatest variety of SIRT foods possible.

SIRT 5-A-DAY PORTION SIZES

Even when choosing foods from the 'Top Ten SIRT Foods' list it can be hard to gauge how much we need to eat for a portion. Is a pinch of turmeric enough? Do I need to eat a whole bowlful of kale? And if I just eat five chocolate biscuits that's my SIRT 5 a day sorted? Right? Not exactly ... but it's not rocket science either. For example, one cup of green tea is a portion, 30g kale (that's a handful to you and me) and ten red grapes constitute a portion. In other words, the amount you would eat as part of a balanced meal is more often than not a sensible portion size.

EXAMPLE MENU 1

Breakfast:
1 cup green tea, 10 red grapes, cereal of your choice
2 of your SIRT 5 a day

• • •

Lunch:
Kale and Stilton soup
3 of your SIRT 5 a day

• • •

Dinner:
Beef and broccoli
2 of your SIRT 5 a day

TOTAL: 7 portions of SIRTs a day

Breakfast:

1 cup green tea, green omelette made with
shallots and parsley

3 of your SIRT 5 a day

• • •

Lunch:

Brie and grape salad lunchbox

4 of your SIRT 5 a day

• • •

Dinner:

Grilled chicken with lemon and olives

2 of your SIRT 5 a day

TOTAL: 9 portions of SIRTs a day

By choosing the foods that are rich natural sources of SIRTs, it is very easy to get your SIRT 5 a day. To boost your SIRTs even more, just add simple snacks like an apple (1 of your SIRT 5 a day), a few squares (30g) of dark chocolate (1 of your SIRT 5 a day) and it soon adds up.

A full list of the most SIRT-rich foods and the relevant portion size for each food is in 'Top SIRT Foods: Quick Reference' (page 60).

More than 5 a day

The SIRT 5 a day is a great way to make sure you are getting enough daily SIRTs and it is a building block you can come back to again and again to make sure you and your family are getting the fantastic benefits of SIRTs.

If you are about to follow The SIRT Diet Plan and want to actively lose weight following the plan, then the SIRT 5 a day is a minimum baseline. As you follow the diet you should be doing everything possible to boost your SIRTs beyond 5 a day, preferably towards 10 a day and beyond. If this sounds hard, then don't worry – all the recipes and details you need to do it are here. The SIRT Diet Plan guides you through it every step of the way with meal planners, shopping tips and sneaky SIRTs to really make sure you are optimising your weight-loss in every way.

THE SIRT DIET PLAN

The SIRT Diet plan is a four-week plan during which you eat SIRT foods at every meal. On the first two days of every week you limit your calories to 800 per day. For the remaining five days of the week you consume up to 1500 calories per day.

Lose up to 14lb on the four-week plan *and* get leaner and fitter as you burn fat, gain muscle and lose weight.

WEEKLY PLAN						
Day 1	Day 2	Day 3	Day 4	Day 5	Day 6	Day 7
JUMP-START	JUMP-START					
800 cals	800 cals	1500 cals	1500 cals	1500 cals	1500 cals	1500 cals
3 light meals	3 light meals	3 meals and 2 snacks	3 meals and 2 snacks	3 meals and 2 snacks	3 meals and 2 snacks	3 meals and 2 snacks
At least 3 portions of SIRTs per meal		At least 3 portions of SIRTs per meal and 1 portion of SIRTs per snack				

EATING SIRT FOODS

There are just two considerations when following the SIRT Diet. Firstly, you must actively seek out SIRT foods and incorporate them into your daily routine. Secondly, you need to show restraint in terms of portion sizes, extra snacks and empty calories. The easiest way to 'show restraint' is to count calories but if you are confident of your ability to track and curb your cravings, then a general awareness of calories rather than vigorous calorie counting should be enough, especially on days that are not jump-start days.

There is one huge advantage of eating SIRT foods that cannot be overlooked. Eating SIRT foods actually controls your appetite, making you less hungry. This is because the SIRT foods convert body fat into energy, reducing your hunger pangs.

You will now be aware of the easiest SIRT foods to fit into your daily life. Is it green tea? Dark chocolate? Red grapes? It is probably all of these and more. This is also where following the meal planners (page 63) and the inspiring SIRT recipes in this book will really help.

You should have a bank of easy SIRT boosters that you can easily reach for if you need a SIRT top-up. Combine SIRT boosters with meals containing one, two or even more portions of SIRTs and you'll find you can easily reach your SIRT targets.

Remember the SIRT 5 a day is a minimum. When you are actively following the SIRT Diet plan – on both jump-start and normal SIRT Diet days – you should aim for at least ten SIRT portions each and every day.

GETTING ENOUGH SIRTS

Are you worried that you can't get enough SIRTs into your diet? Perhaps you have a passionate dislike for kale? Don't worry, there are many different ways to get your daily SIRT requirements. So if there is a food or two you want to avoid, then just steer clear, there are many other options. Have a look through the 'Top SIRT Foods: Quick Reference' (page 60) and see what your favourites (or easy wins) are.

Think about your green vegetables – ideally one to two portions daily. If you don't like the stronger tasting leafy greens, then perhaps plainer broccoli or cauliflower? You only need a handful of parsley (10g) and it has a mild, unobtrusive taste. You could buy a growing pot of parsley from the supermarket and add a portion to your main meal or a salad.

Olive oil and olives – at least one portion a day. Olive oil is such a versatile oil that it can be used in virtually all your cooking. Use extra virgin olive oil in salads and a light and mild version for frying when you don't want an olive-oil flavour.

Onions and apples – at least one portion a day. Raw red onion is great in salads or salsa. Many a main dish starts with lightly sautéed onions. And what could be easier than grabbing an apple as a mid-afternoon snack?

Resveratrol: red wine, red grapes, chocolate – at least two portions a day. Oh the hardship!

Turmeric – at least two portions a week. You only need ½ tsp to get a portion of SIRTs from turmeric. Easy to add to Indian and North African dishes. There are lots of ideas for turmeric in the recipe section of this book.

Oily fish – at least two portions a week. I think you know the drill on this one. Salmon, trout and mackerel all count. Salmon is especially versatile and is very quick to cook. Or try a posh breakfast of smoked salmon and scrambled eggs.

With all these normal everyday foods, it is very easy to increase the amount of SIRTs you eat each day. A few wise decisions will pay huge dividends.

TOP TEN SIRT BOOSTERS

Here are ten easy snacks you can reach for when you need a SIRT top-up.

1 Green tea
1 cup (200ml) • 1 of your SIRT 5 a day • 0 calories

Never, ever, underestimate the healthy SIRT boost that a cup of green tea can give you. Have as many cups as you can per day – I recommend at least two cups. Not only that, the SIRTs in green tea are cumulative so you can get up to four portions of SIRTs daily if you have four cups of green tea or more.

2 Red grapes
10 grapes • 1 of your SIRT 5 a day • 30 calories

A very easy and low-calorie way to get one of your SIRT portions. Keep a punnet or two in the fridge and have a handful at breakfast or lunch or even both!

3 Apples
1 apple • 1 of your SIRT 5 a day • 47 calories

An apple a day really does keep the doctor a way. Reach for an apple as an after-lunch treat. It will help keep sugar cravings at bay too.

4 Cocoa

2 tsp/10g cocoa • **1 of your SIRT 5 a day** • **33 calories**

Try making a chocolate shot with 2 tsp cocoa, 1 tsp sugar and 30ml milk. Mix the cocoa and sugar together with a little boiling water from the kettle to make a smooth paste. Stir in the milk. An (almost) instant chocolate hit with only 68 calories.

5 Olives

6 large black or green olives • **1 of your SIRT 5 a day** • **75 calories**

A versatile snack in the afternoon or a pre-dinner treat. Serve at room temperature to get a fuller flavour.

6 Freshly pressed orange juice

1 small glass (200ml) • **1 of your SIRT 5 a day** • **77 calories**

Squeeze your own or buy fresh orange juice. It must be not from concentrate and with juicy bits.

7 Blackberries

15 blackberries • **1 of your SIRT 5 a day** • **32 calories**

Another easy SIRT fix to keep in your fridge. Available in the supermarket or your nearest hedgerow. Also great as a frozen treat.

8 Dark chocolate 85%

6 squares/20g chocolate • 1 of your SIRT 5 a day
• 125 calories

Get your chocolate hit here! If you prefer 70% dark
chocolate, you'll need 9 squares/30g, which will be
180 calories.

9 Pomegranate seeds

50g/half a small pack • 1 of your SIRT 5 a day
• 50 calories

Easy to obtain while on the go, pomegranate seeds pack
a large SIRT punch and you only need half a 100g pack to
get one of your SIRT portions.

10 Blueberries

25 blueberries (80g) • 1 of your sirt 5 a day • 36 cals

One large handful of blueberries is all you need to get
your SIRT 5 a day.

THE RED WINE QUESTION

For some people, myself included, the idea of a diet that allows any alcohol, particularly one as delicious as red wine, has got to be the best diet ever. There are a few rules to follow when it comes to having a drink (there to make sure you don't go overboard) and you have to stick to red wine as it's the only one that contains resveratrol, one of the most important SIRT bioactives.

One small glass of red wine (125ml) is one of your SIRT 5 a day. I wouldn't recommend any wine on your jump-start days as even a small glass of wine has 120 calories and may encourage you to eat more.

However, on days 3–7, a small glass of red is acceptable, even encouraged, with your evening meal. On days 6 and 7, or whatever days happen to be the weekend, up to 2 small glasses (or 1 large) is allowed. Enjoy the wine knowing it's good for you and helping with your diet, but be aware of how even a small alcoholic drink may affect you. Firstly, it is sometimes hard to resist a second or third glass of wine with the bottle open and the first glass being so tasty. This really isn't allowed on the SIRT diet and is counterproductive. If you find that 1 glass of wine is never enough and willpower is a problem, consider cutting out the wine altogether and getting your SIRTs from other sources. The other tricky concern is does drinking wine make you eat more later in the evening? I find that this can be a problem for me. Even a small glass of wine inspires a 'laissez-faire' attitude and can leave me scurrying for the biscuit tin.

Everyone is different when it comes to their attitude to alcohol and red wine. If red wine is not your favourite tipple, then abstinence (for the diet period at any rate) is the most sure-fire way to lose the pounds. If you like a glass of red, then don't go over the top – 4–5 small glasses a week is the maximum. If you have large wine glasses at home (who doesn't?) then measure 125ml in a measuring jug the first time so you know the correct portion size. A standard wine bottle is 750ml, which is 6 small glasses of wine, so you'll need to make it last. An airtight wine stopper is a good investment as it allows you to keep the wine fresh for several days. I normally stopper the wine after pouring out a glass and then put it away so it is 'out of sight and mind'.

Saying all of this, you should not be discouraged. A delicious glass of red wine is something to savour and enjoy guilt-free on the SIRT Diet.

WHAT ABOUT EXERCISE?

Have a great exercise routine already and have no wish to change it? That's fine. Just carry on as you are, you are off to a great start already. The SIRT Diet gives you plenty of energy (perhaps even more than normal) to follow your normal exercise plan. You should find this is the case even on jump-start days, although maybe skip the marathon that day ...

Not really an exerciser? That's OK too. Obviously as part of any balanced healthy living plan, exercise is always a good idea. At least 30 minutes, three times a week of exercise is a good minimum. However, the SIRT Diet plan isn't about exercise and you don't need to change your current lifestyle to successfully follow the plan.

The beauty of the SIRT diet is that just by eating more SIRT foods you are likely to convert fat to muscle – without changing or increasing your exercise routine *at all*. As well as weight-loss, you will find that you look and feel leaner by the end of the plan and this is due to a reduction in fat and an increase in muscle fibres. This will not be reflected on the scales as muscle is actually slightly heavier than fat. For example, if you lose 10lb on the scales, then by the end of the four-week plan you may have converted another 4lb to muscle. So your total weight-loss is 'only' 10lb, but you will look and feel like you've lost over a stone. Just wait for the compliments to start rolling in.

The only exercise 'guideline' you need for SIRT dieting:

Don't worry about exercise. Just carry
on as you are.

THE JUMP-START

800 CALORIES PER DAY
WITH SIRT FOODS

By restricting calories as well as eating SIRT foods, you will trigger fat-burning genes and get your SIRT diet off to the best possible start.

Eating only 800 calories per day may sound hard, but if you pick your foods carefully – to be filling as well as SIRT-rich – you will not feel more than a little bit hungry. Avoid 'empty' calories in foods like bread and pasta, which will fill you up for an hour or so but leave you starving later on. Instead, pick fibre-rich carbohydrates like oats and beans. Eat some protein and/or fat with every meal as these are the most filling parts of your diet. Chicken, eggs and fish all contain good-quality protein. Dairy, particularly yogurt (the full-fat kind), contains protein and carbs and can be part of a filling and healthy breakfast.

As a rough guide you'll probably want to eat about 200 calories for breakfast, 200 for lunch and 400 for dinner. This enables you to have enough food to curb your hunger pangs during the day and have a 'proper' balanced meal for dinner.

I find that on jump-start days I don't feel hungry during the day – although I do enjoy my food more than normal – and my evening meal is the most important part of the day. The only time I find it hard is later on in the evening when my cravings for unhealthy food are at their highest. I get through them knowing that I can feed my cravings guilt-free with dark chocolate on other days.

It is likely that you will need to keep track of your calories on a jump-start day, especially the first few times you do it. Although it is extremely important to eat plenty of SIRT foods, making sure you don't exceed 800 calories on your jump-start days is the most sure-fire way to lose weight quickly. If you need to take in more SIRTs, try adding green tea, which is calorie free, or add red grapes or other berries, which come in at under 50 calories per portion.

Jump-start breakfast suggestions include: SIRT fruits and yogurt, oat-based cereal + grapes and omelette with green vegetables. All breakfasts should include a cup of green tea.

Jump-start lunch suggestions include: miso soup (either home-made or take-away), young kale salad with chicken or beans, savoy cabbage and bacon soup.

A jump-start dinner should include: protein such as chicken, salmon or prawns, a good source of carbohydrates – think basmati rice, new potatoes in their skin – and plenty of leafy green vegetables and other healthy SIRTs.

Example jump-start day

As a rough guide, you should aim to consume up to 200 calories for breakfast, 200 for lunch and 400 for dinner.

EXAMPLE JUMP-START DAY MENU

Breakfast:
200 calories • 3 portions of SIRTS
Cup of green tea
Fresh SIRT fruit or smoothie

Mid-morning:
Cup of green tea

Lunch:
200 calories • 3 portions of SIRTS
Leafy green salad or miso soup

Dinner:
400 calories • 3 portions of SIRTS
Lean meat such as chicken or fish or tofu/beans
A small portion of good carbs such as brown
rice or new potatoes
Plenty of green vegetables

SIRT DIET DAYS

1500 CALORIES PER DAY
WITH SIRT FOODS

Your primary concern on a 'normal' SIRT diet day is to make sure you get lots and lots of lovely SIRTs.

By now you should know what to choose and what to expect. Add in a few red berries, have a delicious chocolate snack, enjoy a glass of red wine in the evening. Is this the perfect diet? I certainly think so.

There are a few simple rules to follow:

- Avoid empty calories from, for example, white bread, excessive carbs, sugary and refined treats.
- Make sure you get a good balance of protein, carbohydrate and fat in every meal. The meal planners and recipes will help with this if needed.
- Only have SIRT-rich snacks and get most of your energy requirements from your regular meals.

WHAT ABOUT CALORIE COUNTING?

This is up to you. The 1500 calories per day is a guideline daily amount for a woman. A man could eat up to 2000 calories per day and still see similar results. Likewise, if you are currently severely overweight you should cut back to 1800 calories (woman) or 2300 calories (man). Why? Because this calorie restriction will still result in steady and strong weight-loss and will be easier to follow. If a diet is too extreme for your body, then the likelihood of breaking the diet or falling off the wagon is much higher.

If you can manage to accurately calorie count each day, then this is a very good way to follow the diet. It means you are most likely to follow the diet and not tip over into excessive calorie consumption. It's not that hard to count your calories, particularly if you eat similar foods each day and/or use some of the recipes in the book (which are calorie counted per serving). You will quickly find that you know the calorie counts for all regular SIRT foods.

Even if you don't calorie count each day, then it's a good idea to count calories for the first few days so you get a good idea of the amount you should be eating. Now I'm used to the diet, I genuinely find that as long as I resist stupid snacks and stick to three main meals, I easily stay under the target figure.

One of the huge (and I mean *huge*) advantages of eating SIRT foods is that they indisputably curb your appetite, making it much easier to resist snacking between meals.

THE DIET THAT IS IMPOSSIBLE
TO FAIL ...

It's true. You don't 'fail' a diet day if you eat a few too many calories; just get straight back on track the next day. We all know that sometimes we find the cravings impossible to resist. I'm thinking impossible hormones or sharing a bottle of wine with a good friend. Don't let it happen too often and you will be fine.

By far the most important part of the SIRT Diet is eating SIRT foods. Not eaten enough SIRTs today? Then take a look at the list of SIRT boosters and add a few extras in. It's better to have a few extra calories, if they are good SIRT-filled calories, than it is to end the day lacking in SIRTs.

EXAMPLE SIRT DIET DAY

As a rough guide, you should aim to consume up to 300 calories for breakfast, 400 for lunch and 500 for dinner. This leaves 300 calories for snacks, drinks and miscellaneous.

EXAMPLE SIRT DIET DAY MENU

Breakfast:
300 calories • 3 portions of SIRTS
Cup of green tea
Fresh SIRT fruit or smoothie
Healthy cereal or omelette

Mid-morning:
Cup of green tea

Lunch:
400 calories • 3 portions of SIRTS
Salad or soup or lunchbox containing greens and
other SIRT-rich vegetables, onions and olive oil

Mid-afternoon:
optional 100 calorie snack • 1 portion of SIRTS
Dark chocolate or apple

Dinner:
500 calories • 3 portions of SIRTS
Lean meat such as chicken or fish or tofu/beans
Good carbs such as brown rice or new potatoes
Plenty of green vegetables

Evening:
optional 100 calorie snack • 1 portion of SIRTS
Small glass of red wine or red grapes or dark chocolate

LIVING THE DIET

The SIRT Diet is one of the easiest diets to follow. Adjust your mind-set to seek out and enjoy SIRT-rich foods, stock up on your favourites and you are ready to go. An awareness of the best foods to eat, portion size and a dash of willpower are all you need to start losing weight and feel revitalised.

Jump-start days are great for dropping the pounds quickly, but if they don't work for you then just follow the standard SIRT diet (1500 calories) days. You won't lose weight quite as quickly, but you will still lose weight steadily and feel great too!

CHANGE THREE THINGS

The best advice I can give you is to change the way you approach food in just three different ways. By adjusting your mind-set and letting the extra SIRT foods curb your appetite, you will find hunger pangs are reduced and you can follow the SIRT Diet without letting it take over your life.

Firstly, you should think about what are your worst habits. What are the foods, beliefs or bad habits that get in the way of a successful diet? Perhaps like me you're a late-night snacker? A weekend binger? A kids' tea scoffer? Or even a biscuit non-resister?

Change one – break your worst habit

The first thing you need to find is your biggest diet-breaking bad habit. When it comes to over-eating, when are you most likely to buckle? You must work hard to stop this behaviour. This is where willpower comes into play, but also you will find the diet-friendly SIRT foods and proper balanced healthy meals will help enormously.

My worst habit is definitely eating far too much in the evening. This is invariably cheap sweet snacks. I'm not hungry particularly, but my willpower is low and my cravings are high. What do I do to beat this habit? Well the first thing I do is eat a small portion of dark chocolate. I try and eat this slowly and make the treat last as long as possible. I normally find that this fulfils my need for something sweet – although I do have to resist going back to the cupboard for a second helping. If I make it through the evening with only one portion of dark chocolate and nothing else, then I give myself a pat on the back for another diet day achieved successfully.

Here are a few other common bad habits and best advice for breaking the pattern:

- **Eating kids' leftovers**
  Don't want to waste those chips? Carefully cutting off the crusts for fussy children, but find they somehow make their way to your mouth without you realising? I think it's hard for parents to throw good food away and the mindset is that it is preferable to eat them yourself rather than throw them away. This comes from our fear of waste. But just think you might eat 300 to 400 calories of rubbish without even realising. You need to be on guard and aware

of what you might put in your mouth without noticing. Would it really be so bad to throw a few things away? No of course not. Scrape plates straight into the bin when your children have finished and don't leave yourself open to temptation.

- **Unable to turn down biscuits and cakes when offered**
This happens more than we care to mention. Someone in your office brings in a delicious cake and says help yourself. Or even worse they say: 'It'll go to waste if you don't help me eat it.' You're at a friend's house and you are offered a biscuit with your cuppa. How do you say no? Surely only one biscuit or a little slice of cake won't hurt? If this is your biggest weakness then you have to say no. Try not to make a big thing about it. In fact you may find that just saying no with little fuss and just moving on to a different topic may mean that no one really notices. However, you can and should give yourself a big pat on the back because this is one of the hardest things to do.

- **Eating too much when you go out to eat**
Faced with amazing food in a restaurant, it's very easy to eat bread roll, starter, huge main course and an enormous pudding. For a very rare treat then just do it! Life is for living after all. But if it's a habit you do frequently, then one blow-out meal could mean that a whole week of good healthy eating is lost. That is what you have to weigh up. Is it worth it? If you're trying go out for a meal and still be healthy, then go just for a healthy-ish main course without chips or bread and resist the pudding. If you don't have too much carbohydrate, sugar or fried food, then it counts as a success – especially if you eat some SIRT-rich foods too

– although you need to be aware that you probably won't lose weight that day.

- **Weekend splurge**

  Are you good all week, but eat and drink like crazy at the weekend? Does willpower go out of the window because the weekend is a time for having fun? If you are good all week but have a blow-out at the weekend, then you will not lose weight. It's as simple as that. All your hard work during the week is totally lost. Is the pleasure worth the cost? If you need to let your hair down, then choose one aspect to splurge on, but be good on everything else. Want to have a few drinks? Eat a healthy SIRT-rich meal before you start drinking to help resist drink-induced snacking and stick to low-calorie drinks and red wine.

- **Biscuit-tin raider**

  If you've got a biscuit tin for your kids or guests, then it can be hard to resist the temptation when you're feeling run-down. It is *impossible* to forget that it's there. Do you really need a full biscuit tin at home? If you're not due any guests, then maybe empty it all into the bin (this is a job to do in the morning when you're feeling strong) and buy/make SIRT-rich treats when needed.

Remember you are setting out to fix only your *worst* habit. This is the one you should focus on breaking. Try to change your mind-set on just the one thing and everything else should fall into place. Every single day that you don't succumb, give yourself a pat on the back for a job well done.

Change two – drink green tea every day

Love it or loathe it, there's no getting away from it, drinking green tea is an essential part of the SIRT diet.

If you're already a convert to green tea, then congratulations you'll already be reaping the benefits of the extraordinary sirtuins found in green tea. You'll find weight-loss comes more easily, together with a revitalised spirit and glowing skin.

This is for the rest of you. Those of you that think you can follow the SIRT diet without drinking green tea. You simply can't. Even if you dislike it, you're going to need to drink it as it is a core part of the diet.

Why is green tea so vital?

Green tea is the only source of one of the most powerful sirtuin bioactives, catechin. Catechins are so potent that only a small quantity, one small cup, triggers fat metabolism and reduces oxidative stress.

- **Appetite suppressant**
  With a cup or two of green tea inside you, you really notice the difference in terms of hunger pangs. You should find that you don't think about food between meals.
- **A little bit of caffeine**
  A cup of green tea contains about a quarter of the caffeine you'd find in a cup of coffee or half the caffeine you'd find in a cup of black tea. This caffeine is just enough to combine with the catechins to have an even more powerful fat-burning effect. This is the optimum way to convert fat to muscle.

- **More energy**

  Hard to measure but definitely there, the catechins give you a little natural buzz that makes starting the day a smidgeon easier.

- **Cumulative effect**

  The power of green tea keeps on giving and two cups of green tea is better than one cup, three cups is better than two cups, etc. In fact you can get up to four of your SIRT 5 a day from green tea if you drink four or more cups.

- **Zero calorie**

  Green tea is naturally calorie free. It doesn't need sugar or sweetener and gives you energy without the calories.

To prove to myself the benefits of green tea, I have done a little bit of self-experimentation. I conducted the experiment on two consecutive days. On the first, I drank three cups of green tea, one at breakfast and two mid-morning. I also drank my normal quantities of black tea and coffee so that I didn't upset my normal caffeine levels. I ate a small (non-SIRT) breakfast of natural yogurt and honey. On the second day, I drank no green tea but had the same builder's tea and milky coffee and the same breakfast. I was surprised by the difference between the two mornings. The most substantial difference was to my energy levels. I felt noticeably brighter on the green-tea day and was able to get more work done. It felt like a little extra zing in my step, different and discernible from my standard morning caffeine buzz. The second difference was my hunger. I really didn't feel hungry all morning on the green-tea day and didn't think about food at all until lunchtime, despite my insubstantial breakfast.

On the day when I didn't drink green tea, I was hungry and my stomach was rumbling before 11am.

This was enough to convert me to drinking green tea, even though I didn't like it much at first. If you're feeling brave or don't quite trust my results, try a little experiment yourself. You won't believe the difference.

Learning to love green tea

A lot of people say that they really dislike the taste of green tea. I agree it's not a taste that most people will instantly like – especially if you've never tried it before. But a bit of perseverance pays dividends here. The first cup may be horrible, the fourth just doable, the tenth nearly enjoyable and by the second week of regular drinking it should be pleasant and refreshing. I am a total convert now. If you find it truly difficult, start with two cups a day: one before or with breakfast and one mid-morning. Pour a small weak cup of tea and wait for it to cool to easy drinking temperature. Then just drink it quickly like medicine. Treat it like a necessary evil if required, and I promise you it will get easier.

If you find the tea too 'grassy' tasting, then try white tea. This is a little bit more expensive but has a cleaner taste. It is still my favourite. You will also notice a difference in brands. If you don't like one brand, try another as they are all subtly different. If you pay a bit more for a quality brand then you should get a fresher taste. There are also several flavoured green teas that might turn out to be 'the one': mint, lemon and jasmine are all common and there are many wonderful-sounding green fruit teas available too. All green and white teas contain the wonderful catechins.

The tea ritual for people that hate tea rituals

Boil the kettle and then leave for 30 seconds to a minute so that it goes 'off the boil'. Pour over the tea leaves or tea bag. Leave to brew for 2–4 minutes, depending on the brew strength required. Start off with a short brewing time and build up gradually. Loose leaf tea is really tasty but you need a special teapot, so if you're happy with teabags, stick to them. Also a glass or delicate china cup complements the subtle flavour.

Recycling your teabags (twice) or tea leaves (up to four times) is positively encouraged. The second cup often tastes even nicer than the first. This is also a great way to make your tea go a lot further and be significantly cheaper per cup.

What about my normal tea and coffee?

If like me, you have a standard routine for tea and/or coffee in the morning that you would hate to break, then don't worry. If these things bring you pleasure then you shouldn't stop them. You should add your green tea on as an extra, rather than deprive yourself. As long as you have at least two cups of green tea a day then your other drinks are up to you.

Change three – eat three balanced meals a day

A balanced meal contains plenty of SIRTs, protein, fat and a small amount of carbohydrate. We tend to think of meat as the primary source of protein, of cheese and fried foods as being loaded with fat (and therefore bad) and carbohydrates being predominantly bread, pasta, potatoes and rice. It's not quite that black and white and there are some foods or food combinations that give you a great balance of protein, fat and carbohydrate. These foods are 'naturally balanced', meaning you can reduce the need to always eat meat for protein and 100% carbs like pasta.

Naturally balanced foods containing protein, fat and carbs

1 Natural yogurt
2 Beans of all varieties, including baked beans
3 Lentils
4 Tofu
5 Dark chocolate

If you are vegetarian, my top food combination is brown rice and lentils – as seen in the One-pot Curry and Rice (page 180) – as this gives a perfect balance of protein, fat and carbs, is exceptionally filling and gives you the essential amino acids that are normally only found in red meat.

Your carbohydrate consumption should never be more than 40% per meal, which means that often you will need to up your intake of fats and protein at mealtimes. This can seem counterintuitive and may mean you are eating slightly smaller portions. But with fewer empty calories you will naturally eat less and stay fuller for much longer.

The simplest way to cut down on carbs is to reduce the amount of bread and pasta you eat. With a sandwich or pasta dish you could easily be eating 80% carbs or more. Instead the majority of your carbs should be the ones that are naturally occurring in fruit and vegetables. Fruit contains carbs in the form of fruit sugar or fructose. Fruit is encouraged as a healthy source of carbs and many fruits have the bonus of being SIRT-rich. Restrained portions of fibre-rich carbohydrates such as brown basmati rice (recommended portion size: 125g cooked rice) and new potatoes in their skins (recommended portion size: 180g new potatoes) are the best carbs to eat as part of a balanced meal.

Unbeatable food combinations

These combinations include a great balance of protein/fat/carbs and contain a good source of SIRTs too.

1 Natural yogurt with berries
2 Rocket salad with beans and cheese
3 Young leaf kale with lentils and chicken
4 Miso soup with noodles
5 Black-bean brownies

TOP TIPS FOR SIRT DIETING

Use this handy guide to getting started with top tips tailored to you.

IF YOU WORK IN AN OFFICE

- A little bit of preparation in the morning pays huge dividends. Having a pre-prepared tasty lunch will be something to really look forward to.
- Buy some green tea bags for the office so you can top up on green tea while you work.
- Try not to be tempted by extra treats and snacks when you pop out to the shops.
- If you need to buy lunch once in a while, go for a healthy green salad containing leafy greens and lean protein such as chicken or fish.
- On a jump-start day buy (or bring in a flask of) miso soup. Both Yo! Sushi and Pret do a good miso soup to take away.

IF YOU'RE FEEDING A FAMILY

- Keep your fridge stacked with blueberries and red grapes: a SIRT booster for you and a healthy snack for your kids.
- Always cook with olive oil where possible and sneak onions and green vegetables into family meals as much as you can.
- If you struggle to get your kids to eat salads, make a big salad with lots of SIRT-rich green leaves and an olive-oil dressing. The kids can pick and choose the bits they eat and you get all your lovely SIRTs.
- Be firm and never allow yourself to eat your children's crusts or leftovers.
- Buy individual packs of biscuits or treats for your children instead of a tempting family-sized pack. Then buy a 70%/85% chocolate bar and keep it just for you.

IF YOU'RE SINGLE

- Make a batch of SIRT-rich meals, refrigerate one or two and freeze the others. This way you've always got an easy SIRT meal waiting for you.
- Save your red wine for when you go out and don't drink at home.
- Have a secret stash of dark chocolate ready for emergencies.
- Don't be tempted by a take-away; it's so easy to over-eat.
- Bags of prepared kale, spinach or rocket are great to have to hand. Add them to any meal for an instant SIRT booster.

IF YOU'RE A VEGETARIAN

- Eat beans, soya beans and tofu to boost your protein intake and SIRT levels.
- Paneer is a great cooking cheese made from semi-skimmed milk that works well in many dishes, not just Indian food.
- Remember combining brown rice and lentils gives you the same essential amino acids you find in red meat.
- Peanuts or peanut-based snacks will keep you full, provide SIRTs and give you extra protein.
- Experiment with spicy options for added flavour. Vegetable curries are fabulous. Try Fresh saag paneer (page 173) or Kale, edamame and tofu curry (page 201).

IF YOU ARE A SERIAL DIET FAILURE

- Remember the most important thing is to eat enough SIRT foods. If you've eaten your daily allowance your day is a success – even if you've had a few extra calories.
- Green tea is your diet friend. It could be the difference between this diet and all the others. Learn to love it ... it may change your life.
- Don't worry about jump-start days. If they're too hard, give them up and stick to the SIRTs. You will still lose weight.
- Concentrate on your one bad habit. If you break one you are well on the way to a healthier you.
- It really is impossible to 'fail' this diet.

IF YOU'RE DIETING AS A COUPLE

- Clear the cupboards of all cakes, biscuits and sweet treats. Remove beer from the house.
- A little bit of competitive spirit should spur you both on and make you less likely to cheat.
- Enjoy a glass of red wine together at the end of a hard day.
- Consider buying a dark chocolate bar each so you don't argue over who's eaten what.
- Make a pot of green tea instead of a cup and always make sure there's enough for your partner. You'll both end up drinking more tea.

SHOPPING FOR
THE SIRT DIET

There's a few things that I find I buy time and time again now I'm following the SIRT Diet. Some are obvious – you just need to stock up on more than usual – but some you may not have heard of before.

1 Red grapes

I just can't get enough of these. I used to buy green grapes for the kids, but now I buy two to three punnets of these a week. Everyone in the house eats them. I make sure that I get the delicious SIRTs either for breakfast or when I need a little sweet hit. The kids love them too and I'm happy knowing they are eating something tasty and healthy.

2 Baby kale leaves

This is a brilliant product that I didn't know existed until recently. Save the big chewy kale for soups and stews and search out baby leaf kale in the salad aisle. Great in salads or lightly steamed, this kale is absolutely bursting with SIRTs and is a must-have SIRT diet purchase.

3 Frozen soya beans

Again, not one I would normally have in my freezer, but I have learnt to love these amazing versatile beans. Cheap and cheerful and located next to the frozen peas in the supermarket. They are quick to cook and have a wonderful nutty flavour. Use them in salads and stir-frys.

4 70% and 85% dark chocolate

There are several brands available, with slightly different flavours. My favourite is Green & Black's. Make sure it is not cooking or Belgian chocolate.

5 Red onion and shallots

As well as normal white onions for cooking, seek out red onions and shallots, which have even more SIRTs than white onions. Red onions work particularly well in salads and hold their shape more than other onions. You can substitute shallots for white onions in pretty much any recipe.

6 Turmeric, mild chilli powder and ground cumin

If you're not used to spices, try this trio, featuring the SIRT-rich turmeric, which add a mild and rich flavour to any dish. For two people you'll need approximately ½ tsp ground turmeric, 1 tsp mild chilli powder and ½ tsp ground cumin.

7 Tofu

Tofu can be found in the vegetarian/specialist aisle of any supermarket. Even if it's not your favourite, consider adding it to any dish to boost the protein and SIRT content. Use in any Chinese or spiced dish, or add to a prawn dish to increase the SIRT content without adding many calories.

8 Capers

A much overlooked condiment. Adds a salty tang to any sauce or salad. Adding just 1 tablespoon to a dish gives you an extra 1 of your SIRT 5 a day. Capers make a delicious and very SIRT-rich salad dressing: 1 tbsp capers, juice of ½ lemon, 1 tbsp extra virgin olive oil, 1 tsp American mustard and lots of salt and pepper.

9 Light and mild olive oil

Adding mild olive oil to your repertoire as well as normal and extra virgin olive oil, allows you to use olive oil in sweet dishes as well as savoury. Mild olive oil does not add the distinctive olive taste to a dish, so is great for Asian dishes too. Olive oil is so much healthier and more natural than other oils. Olive oil is now my preferred oil in virtually all cooking.

10 Belgian dark chocolate chips

These delicious chocolate chips are 70% cocoa solids and, being Belgian, they are less bitter than other dark chocolate. Great for baking or grab a handful for a little chocolate treat.

SIRT FLAVOUR FIXERS

The food that you eat on the SIRT Diet should never ever be bland. If your dinner doesn't delight your taste buds, then you are far more likely to want to eat something 'bad' afterwards. There are many simple ways to do this without adding to the calories. As a bonus you can sometimes add in a few extra SIRTs too.

Salt and freshly ground black pepper

I know this sounds basic, but it makes such a difference that it is worth a special mention. I don't tend to include much salt while I am cooking, but I always check the seasoning before I serve. Sometimes a little grind of salt will transform a dish. If you taste a sauce and you can't really taste any of the individual flavours, then you may have under-salted. Add a little at a time as over-salted food is even worse.

Likewise, I don't think there are many dishes that are not enhanced by a little freshly ground black pepper.

Onions and garlic

When you think about it, onions and garlic are ingredients you wouldn't want to be without in sauces and casseroles. Onions can be cooked slowly for a deep flavour – try sprinkling with salt to bring out their natural sweetness – or more quickly to get a caramelized golden onion with more bite. Onions and garlic both add SIRTs to a dish. Raw red onions add the most SIRTs, then shallots, then white onions and finally garlic. Garlic has only a very small amount of SIRTs, but adds a lot of flavour and at only 4 calories a clove, I like to use it liberally. You don't need much olive oil to fry onions and garlic – 1 teaspoon of olive oil for 1 onion is normally enough. For best results, heat the oil on a medium heat and toss in the onion when hot. Fry for 2 minutes before adding any garlic (it needs less time to cook), turning the heat down to the lowest setting and putting the lid on the pan. A lidded pan allows the onion and garlic to steam as well as fry, retaining more SIRTs and cooking quicker. Cook with the lid on for 5 minutes for perfectly cooked onion and garlic.

Parsley

Fresh parsley really enhances any dish – especially traditional British dishes and anything European, Mediterranean or North African. You don't need much to get 1 of your SIRT 5 a day either. 10g is a portion of parsley, which roughly translates as a small handful. The benefits of adding parsley to a dish are subtle. It doesn't change the flavour, as some herbs and spices are wont to do, but it significantly enhances it. I like to buy a pot of parsley from the supermarket, which lasts a lot longer than cut parsley. If you look after your growing pot by placing it in a sunny location and watering daily, a large pot of parsley can last up to a month.

Turmeric and other spices

Although turmeric is the only spice to add SIRTs to a dish, it is heightened when combined with other spices such as paprika and cumin.

Try these rough and ready country-based flavour combinations to add to any meat or vegetarian dish. These are enough to serve two people – adjust accordingly for smaller or larger meals.

Indian classic: ½ tsp ground turmeric, ½ tsp ground cumin, ½ tsp ground coriander, 1 tsp chilli powder

Indian sweet: 1 tsp ground turmeric, ¼ tsp ground cinnamon, ¼ tsp ground cloves, 1 tsp mild chilli powder, 1 tsp paprika

Indian hot: ½ tsp ground turmeric, ½ tsp cayenne pepper, 1 tsp chilli powder, ½ tsp ground cumin, 1 fresh chilli (chopped, seeds in if you like it really hot)

North African: ¼ tsp ground cinnamon, ½ tsp ground turmeric, 2 strands saffron, ¼ tsp ground ginger, 1 tsp dried mixed herbs, juice of ½ lemon

Mexican: ½ tsp mild chilli powder, ½ tsp ground coriander, juice of 1 lime, fresh parsley and coriander

NEW ESSENTIALS SHOPPING LIST

Fruit and veg

Apples

Red grapes

Blackcurrants

Blueberries

Blackberries

Oranges and satsumas

Lemons

Limes

Pomegranate seeds

Baby kale

Young spinach

Watercress leaves

Broccoli

Rocket

Red onions

Shallots

Meat and fish

Salmon fillets

Chilled and frozen

Tofu

Olives

Smoked salmon

Frozen soya beans

Frozen mixed berries

Herbs and spices

Ground turmeric

Chilli powder

Ground cumin

Fresh parsley

Store cupboard

Olive oil

Extra virgin olive oil

Mild olive oil

Soy sauce

Capers

Anchovies

Ready-to-eat kidney beans

Ready-to-eat cannellini beans

70% dark chocolate

85% dark chocolate

Unsweetened cocoa powder

Belgian dark chocolate chips

Green or white tea

Matcha green tea powder

WHEN YOU'RE OUT AND ABOUT

SNACKING ON THE GO

- **Wasabi peas**
  Delicious and filling and sometimes really, really hot! Although a little high in calories, wasabi peas are preferable to crisps and nuts. Wasabi and Japanese horseradish both contain SIRTs, so you would also get half a portion of your SIRT 5 a day.

- **Plain roasted and salted peanuts**
  A bit too calorific for everyday eating, yet peanuts contain SIRTs, are rich in protein and fat and are surprisingly filling. Go for salted peanuts as these do not have added sugar and flavourings. A small snack pack can give you enough energy to last for up to 4 hours.

- **Mini chocolate bars**
  You'll find these mini chocolate bars or dark chocolate squares on the counter in most coffee shops. One is approximately one of your SIRT 5 a day and hits the sweet spot nicely.

- **Green tea**
  It's surprising how many places serve green tea nowadays: all the coffee shops and many restaurants and cafes. Feel totally calorie and guilt-free having one of these.

- **Kale crisps**

  Look in the 'posh crisps' section for these delicious crisps. Not as healthy as simple kale, but a fab snack that gives you an extra ½ of your SIRT 5 a day.

- **Chocolate brownie**

  Not exactly the perfect snack, but brownies tend to have a high cocoa content so are more SIRT diet friendly than other cakes and treats.

LUNCHTIME

If you're trying to catch a quick bite to eat at lunchtime, then you still need to stay healthy, get some SIRTs in and stay away from the sandwiches.

A salad is perhaps the most obvious choice. Choose a salad with rich dark leaves like spinach or watercress as these are the most SIRT-rich. Make sure there is plenty of filling protein in the form of chicken or (even better from a SIRT point of view) salmon. A salad containing beans or edamame will have the double advantage of being extra filling and SIRT diet friendly.

Another option is soup. Miso soup or ramen are good choices and can be bought 'to go' from some restaurants like Yo! Sushi or Wagamama. Cabbage, spinach or watercress soup are all good choices, as are bean soups. Mixed-bean soup is particularly warming and filling on a cold winter's day.

For dessert, stick to SIRT-rich fruits like berries, red grapes or an apple. Many shops also sell tiny bars of chocolate, which make a great accompaniment to a cup of green tea.

CHOOSING A RESTAURANT

Eating out needn't be too difficult as long as you pick your restaurant and food carefully. The restaurant styles best suited to the SIRT way of eating are those that cook with plenty of fresh, seasonal vegetables. For that reason, a traditional British restaurant, particularly one specialising in fresh local produce, is likely to be a good bet. For similar reasons, French bistros and Spanish tapas restaurants are also a good place to go. When you go to a restaurant, throwing caution to the wind is probably not a good idea – you could dispose of a week's worth of healthy eating in one sitting! Instead follow a simple mantra of more SIRTs and fewer empty calories. In practice this will mean looking out for the dishes with plenty of green vegetables, salads or oily fish. A SIRT-rich starter such as a plate of olives is definitely allowed, but steer clear of the bread roll. For dessert you can probably find something with chocolate and/or berries, but be aware that a large creamy pudding may contain up to 1000 calories...so choose wisely.

Restaurants to avoid are any take-away-style outlets, as these will be fatty, calorific and lacking in SIRTs. Also on the no-go list are curry houses (not enough SIRTs), pasta and pizza parlours (too many carbs) and your local chip shop (fat and carbs).

TOP SIRT FOODS: QUICK REFERENCE

The portion sizes listed below give an approximation of how much of the foodstuff you need to consume to get 1 of your SIRT 5 a day. Remember you should aim for at least 5 SIRT portions every day.

Vegetables	
Kale	30g
Spinach	50g
Watercress	50g
Rocket	50g
Parsley	10g
Red onion	¼ (45g)
Shallot	1 (50g)
White onion	½ (90g)
Savoy cabbage	150g
Pak choi	100g
Broccoli	100g
Cauliflower	150g
Soya beans/edamame	80g
Tofu	80g
Olives	6 large (50g)

Fruit	
Red grapes	10 grapes (50g)
Blackcurrants	30g
Redcurrants	50g
Pomegranate seeds	50g
Pomegranate juice	100ml
Blackberries	100g
Blueberries	80g
Strawberries	100g
Raspberries	100g
Apple	1 large (120g)
Apple juice, fresh	200ml
Orange	1 large (140g)
Orange juice, fresh	200ml
Lemon	Juice of 2
Lime	Juice of 2

Fish	
Salmon	130g (1 fillet)
Anchovy fillets	20g (2 fillets)
Trout	130g (1 fillet)
Sardines	50g (2 fillets)

Other

Ground turmeric	½ tsp (2g)
Extra virgin olive oil	1 tsp (5ml)
Olive oil	1 tbsp (15ml)
Red wine	200ml
Soy sauce	2 tbsp (30ml)
Cocoa powder	2 tsp (10g)
Dark chocolate (70%)	30g
Green tea	1 cup
Matcha green tea powder	1 tsp (5g)
Kidney beans	120g (½ drained can)
Butter beans	120g
Black-eyed beans	120g
Black beans	120g
Cannellini beans	120g
Haricot beans	120g
Peanuts	100g
Capers	1 tbsp (10g)

COMPLETE FOUR-WEEK PLAN

Use this detailed guide to organize your food choices for the week. This guide is intended to be as practical as possible, with quick weekday dinner choices and more complex meals and baking at the weekend. If a dish makes several portions, then where possible you'll be able to keep leftovers and have them the next day. As you become more confident with the SIRT way of eating, feel free to replace a meal with a similar dish. I have tried to accommodate a really good balance of fat, protein and good carbs as well as plenty of SIRT-rich foods. There's also a few snacks and cakes for when you need a treat.

WEEK 1 MEAL PLANNER

Monday	Tuesday	Wednesday	Thursday
JUMP-START	JUMP-START		
GREEN TEA			
Blueberry smoothie (p. 81) 160 cals 1 of your SIRT 5 a day	SIRT fruit salad (p. 78) 172 cals 3 of your SIRT 5 a day	Green omelette (p. 83) 234 cals 2½ of your SIRT 5 a day	Choc chip granola (p. 84) with 150ml milk 323 cals ½ of your SIRT 5 a day
GREEN TEA			
French country salad (p. 123) 245 cals 5 of your SIRT 5 a day	Parsley soup (p. 157) 232 cals 3 of your SIRT 5 a day	Brie and grape salad with honey dressing (p. 138) 378 cals 4 of your SIRT 5 a day	Sesame chicken salad (p. 133) 465 cals 4 of your SIRT 5 a day
		1 apple 47 cals 1 of your SIRT 5 a day	100g blackberries 32 cals 1 of your SIRT 5 a day
Teriyaki salmon with Chinese vegetables (p. 178) 354 cals 2½ of your SIRT 5 a day	Mini turkey burgers with parsley salad (p. 186) 363 cals 3 of your SIRT 5 a day	Turmeric prawns (p. 166) 414 cals 3 of your SIRT 5 a day	One-pot curry and rice (p. 180) 347 cals 2 of your SIRT 5 a day
1 apple 47 cals 1 of your SIRT 5 a day	Handful (80g) blueberries 36 cals 1 of your SIRT 5 a day	Small glass (125ml) of red wine and 30g 70% dark choc 300 cals 2 of your SIRT 5 a day	Green tea and choc chip loaf (p. 238) 313 cals 1 of your SIRT 5 a day
806 calories **11½ SIRT portions**	**803 calories** **12 SIRT portions**	**1373 calories** **14½ SIRT portions**	**1480 calories** **10½ SIRT portions**

Friday	Saturday	Sunday
(1 of your SIRT 5 a day)		
Blackcurrant and oat yogurt swirl (p. 82) 241 cals 1½ of your SIRT 5 a day	Very green juice (p. 75) 100g natural yogurt, 1tsp honey, 10 red grapes 346 cals 2 of your SIRT 5 a day	Apple pancakes with blackcurrant compote (p. 87) 340 cals 1½ of your SIRT 5 a day
(1 of your SIRT 5 a day)		
One-pot curry and rice (p. 180) 347 cals 2 of your SIRT 5 a day	Pomegranate, feta and walnut salad (p. 128) 340 cals 3 of your SIRT 5 a day	Mexican chicken soup (p. 147) 361 cals 2 of your SIRT 5 a day
30g 70% dark choc 180 cals 1 of your SIRT 5 a day	Chocolate shot (p. 100) 68 cals 1 of your SIRT 5 a day	1 apple 47 cals 1 of your SIRT 5 a day
Sticky pork with apple (p. 207) with 180g new potatoes 449 cals 2 of your SIRT 5 a day	Kale and tomato pasta (p. 179) 520 cals 5 of your SIRT 5 a day	Beef in red wine with kale mashed potato (p. 202) 651 cals 4 of your SIRT 5 a day
Green tea and choc chip loaf (p. 238) 313 cals 1 of your SIRT 5 a day	Large glass (175ml) of red wine 168 cals 1½ of your SIRT 5 a day	6 squares (20g) 85% dark choc 125 cals 1 of your SIRT 5 a day
1530 calories 9½ SIRT portions	**1442 calories 14½ SIRT portions**	**1524 calories 11½ SIRT portions**

WEEK 2 MEAL PLANNER

Monday	Tuesday	Wednesday	Thursday
JUMP-START	JUMP-START		
GREEN TEA			
Raspberry and blackcurrant jelly (p. 86) 76 cals 2 of your SIRT 5 a day	Raspberry and blackcurrant jelly (p. 86) 76 cals 2 of your SIRT 5 a day	Kale savoury muffin (p. 234) and glass of fresh orange 270 cals 2 of your SIRT 5 a day	Kale savoury muffin (p. 234) and glass of fresh orange 270 cals 2 of your SIRT 5 a day
GREEN TEA			
Mexican chicken soup (p. 147) 361 cals 2 of your SIRT 5 a day	Garlic butter chicken with rocket salad (p. 124) 334 cals 3 of your SIRT 5 a day	Garlic butter chicken with rocket salad (p. 124) 334 cals 3 of your SIRT 5 a day	Savoy cabbage and bacon soup (p. 150) 296 cal 2 of your SIRT 5 a day
		50g pomegranate seeds 50 cals 1 of your SIRT 5 a day	30g 75% dark chocolate 180 cals 1 of your SIRT 5 a day
Smoked salmon and new potato salad (p. 130) 348 cals 4 of your SIRT 5 a day	Quick vegetable stir-fry with black-bean sauce (p. 168) 343 cals 4 of your SIRT 5 a day	Soy-glazed salmon (p. 170) with 125g cooked rice and 80g broccoli 508 cals 2½ of your SIRT 5 a day	Hot chipolata and redcurrant salad (p. 136) with 180g new potatoes 455 cals 3 of your SIRT 5 a day
10 red grapes 33 cals 1 of your SIRT 5 a day	Handful (80g) blueberries 36 cals 1 of your SIRT 5 a day	Small glass (125ml) of red wine and 30g 70% dark choc 300 cals 2 of your SIRT 5 a day	Apple and blackberry cake (p. 232) 249 cals ½ of your SIRT 5 a day
818 calories **11 SIRT portions**	**789 calories** **12 SIRT portions**	**1462 calories** **12½ SIRT portions**	**1450 calories** **10½ SIRT portions**

Friday	Saturday	Sunday
(1 of your SIRT 5 a day)		
Very green juice (p. 75) 206 cals 1 of your SIRT 5 a day	Blackcurrant and oat yogurt swirl (p. 82) 241 cals 1½ of your SIRT 5 a day	Blackcurrant and oat yogurt swirl (p. 82) 241 cals 1½ of your SIRT 5 a day
(1 of your SIRT 5 a day)		
Savoy cabbage and bacon soup (p. 150) 296 cal 2 of your SIRT 5 a day	French country salad (p. 123) 245 cals 5 of your SIRT 5 a day	French country salad (p. 123) 245 cals 5 of your SIRT 5 a day
Kale savoury muffin (p. 234) 193 cals 1 of your SIRT 5 a day	1 apple 47 cals 1 of your SIRT 5 a day	1 orange 73 cals 1 of your SIRT 5 a day
Chicken and watercress pie (p. 199) with 80g broccoli 564 calories of your SIRT 5 a day	Chicken and watercress pie (p. 199) with 80g broccoli 564 calories 3 of your SIRT 5 a day	Quick-fried beef with salsa verde (p. 176) with 180g new potatoes 481 cals 2 of your SIRT 5 a day
Apple and blackberry cake (p. 232) 249 cals ½ of your SIRT 5 a day	Chocolate and blackberry mini pavlovas (p. 216) 428 cals 2 of your SIRT 5 a day	Chocolate and blackberry mini pavlovas (p. 216) 428 cals 2 of your SIRT 5 a day
1508 calories **9½ SIRT portions**	**1525 calories** **14½ SIRT portions**	**1468 calories** **13½ SIRT portions**

Monday	Tuesday	Wednesday	Thursday
JUMP-START	JUMP-START		
GREEN TEA			
SIRT fruit salad (p. 78) 172 cals 3 of your SIRT 5 a day	Egg florentine (p. 110) 215 cals 2 of your SIRT 5 a day	Green omelette (p. 83) 234 cals 2½ of your SIRT 5 a day	Blueberry smoothie (p. 81) 160 cals 1 of your SIRT 5 a day
GREEN TEA			
No-cook falafel lunchbox (p. 113) 387 cals 4 of your SIRT 5 a day	No-cook falafel lunchbox (p. 113) 387 cals 4 of your SIRT 5 a day	No-cook falafel lunchbox (p. 113) 387 cals 4 of your SIRT 5 a day	No-cook falafel lunchbox (p. 113) 387 cals 4 of your SIRT 5 a day
		30g 70% dark choc 180 cals 1 of your SIRT 5 a day	3 chocolate and lime truffles (p. 227) 192 cals 1 of your SIRT 5 a day
Fragrant Asian hotpot (p. 175) 185 cals 1½ of your SIRT 5 a day	Fragrant Asian hotpot (p. 175) 185 cals 1½ of your SIRT 5 a day	Cheesy greens pasta bake (p. 205) 526 cals 2 of your SIRT 5 a day	Creamy fish pie (p. 189) with 180g new potatoes and 80g broccoli 532 cals 3 of your SIRT 5 a day
Chocolate shot (p. 100) 68 cals 1 of your SIRT 5 a day	10 red grapes 33 cals 1 of your SIRT 5 a day	3 chocolate and lime truffles (p. 227) 192 cals 1 of your SIRT 5 a day	Chocolate cupcake with matcha icing (p. 236) 234 cals 1 of your SIRT 5 a day
812 calories 11½ SIRT portions	**820 calories 10½ SIRT portions**	**1519 calories 12½ SIRT portions**	**1505 calories 12 SIRT portions**

Friday	Saturday	Sunday
(1 of your SIRT 5 a day)		
SIRT fruit salad (p. 78) 172 cals 3 of your SIRT 5 a day	Chocolate cupcake with matcha icing (p. 236) 234 cals 1 of your SIRT 5 a day	Chocolate cupcake with matcha icing (p. 236) 234 cals 1 of your SIRT 5 a day
(1 of your SIRT 5 a day)		
Spicy butternut squash and kale soup (p. 152) 340 cals 2½ of your SIRT 5 a day	Spicy butternut squash and kale soup (p. 152) 340 cals 2½ of your SIRT 5 a day	Mini turkey burgers with parsley salad (p. 186) 363 cals 3 of your SIRT 5 a day
3 chocolate and lime truffles (p. 227) 192 cals 1 of your SIRT 5 a day	Crunchy fried olives (p. 98) 343 cals 2½ of your SIRT 5 a day	Crunchy fried olives (p. 98) 343 cals 2½ of your SIRT 5 a day
Creamy fish pie (p. 189) with 180g new potatoes and 80g broccoli 532 cals 3 of your SIRT 5 a day	Chinese-style pork with pak choi (p. 196) 377 cals 2 of your SIRT 5 a day	Turmeric prawns (p. 166) 414 cals 3 of your SIRT 5 a day
Chocolate cupcake with matcha icing (p. 236) 234 cals of your SIRT 5 a day	Large glass (175ml) of red wine 168 cals 1½ of your SIRT 5 a day	Large glass (175ml) of red wine 168 cals 1½ of your SIRT 5 a day
1470 calories **12½ SIRT portions**	**1462 calories** **11½ SIRT portions**	**1522 calories** **13 SIRT portions**

Monday	Tuesday	Wednesday	Thursday
JUMP-START	JUMP-START		
GREEN TEA			
Chocolate matcha energy balls (p. 102) 111 cals 1 of your SIRT 5 a day	Chocolate matcha energy balls (p. 102) 111 cals 1 of your SIRT 5 a day	Very green juice (p. 75) 100g natural yogurt, 1 tsp honey 310 cals 1 of your SIRT 5 a day	Grape and melon juice (p. 77), Cocoa and grape cereal bar (p. 231) 286 cals 2½ of your SIRT 5 a day
GREEN TEA			
LA Green salad (p. 135) 304 cals 2½ of your SIRT 5 a day	Greens in curried broth (p. 158) 130 cals 3 of your SIRT 5 a day	Mexican chicken soup (p. 147) 361 cals 2 of your SIRT 5 a day	Mexican chicken soup (p. 147) 361 cals 2 of your SIRT 5 a day
	20g 85% dark chocolate 125 cals 1 of your SIRT 5 a day	10 red grapes 33 cals 1 of your SIRT 5 a day	20g 85% dark chocolate 125 cals 1 of your SIRT 5 a day
Mini turkey burgers with parsley salad (p. 186) 363 cals 3 of your SIRT 5 a day	Roast chicken and kale salad with peanut dressing (p. 139) 383 cals 2 of your SIRT 5 a day	Kale, edamame and tofu curry (p. 201) with 125g cooked brown rice 501 cals 2½ of your SIRT 5 a day	Teriyaki salmon with Chinese vegetables (p. 178) 354 cals 2 ½ of your SIRT 5 a day
Pomegranate and blueberry ice (p. 220) 55 cals 1½ of your SIRT 5 a day	Pomegranate and blueberry ice (p. 220) 55 cals 1½ of your SIRT 5 a day	Small glass (125ml) of red wine and 30g 70% dark choc 300 cals 2 of your SIRT 5 a day	Extreme chocolate mousse (p. 218) 375 cals 1½ of your SIRT 5 a day
833 calories **10 SIRT portions**	**804 calories** **10½ SIRT portions**	**1505 calories** **10½ SIRT portions**	**1501 calories** **11½ SIRT portions**

Friday	Saturday	Sunday
(1 of your SIRT 5 a day)		
Grape and melon juice (p. 77, Cocoa and grape cereal bar (p. 231) 286 cals 2½ of your SIRT 5 a day	Apple pancakes with blackcurrant compote (p. 87) 340 cals 1½ of your SIRT 5 a day	Green tea smoothie (p. 79) 183 cals 1 of your SIRT 5 a day
(1 of your SIRT 5 a day)		
Mexican salsa with Wensleydale and cucumber pittas (p. 116) 324 cals 1½ of your SIRT 5 a day	Greek salad skewers (p. 109) 306 cals 3½ of your SIRT 5 a day	Brie and grape salad with honey dressing (p. 138) 383 cals 3 of your SIRT 5 a day
6 large olives 75 cals 1 of your SIRT 5 a day	Cocoa and grape cereal bar (p. 231) 161 cals ½ of your SIRT 5 a day	20g 85% dark chocolate 125 cals 1 of your SIRT 5 a day
Chicken with pesto crust (p. 198) 180g new potatoes and 80g broccoli 484 calories 2½ of your SIRT 5 a day	Tandoori chicken and peas (p. 185) 461 cals 4 of your SIRT 5 a day	Beef in red wine with kale mashed potato (p. 202) 651 cals 4 of your SIRT 5 a day
Extreme chocolate mousse (p. 218) 375 cals 1½ of your SIRT 5 a day	Blackcurrant ripple meringues (p. 213) 229 cals 1 of your SIRT 5 a day	Large glass (175ml) of red wine 168 cals 1½ of your SIRT 5 a day
1496 calories 10 SIRT portions	**1497 calories 12½ SIRT portions**	**1510 calories 12½ SIRT portions**

BREAKFAST CHOICES

To start the day right, a cup (or three) of green tea is a very good place to begin. Green tea, a fresh orange or a handful of red grapes, together with a light breakfast of your choice, will set you up just right for the day. If you like the extra spring in your step that a smoothie or juice gives you, there are some fantastic SIRT-rich ones here to try.

●　●　●

Very Green Juice

Summer Watermelon Juice

Grape and Melon Juice

SIRT Fruit Salad

Green Tea Smoothie

Kale and Blackcurrant Smoothie

Blueberry Smoothie

Blackcurrant and Oat Yogurt Swirl

Green Omelette

Choc Chip Granola

Raspberry and Blackcurrant Jelly

Apple Pancakes with Blackcurrant Compote

Very Green Juice

206 calories

1
of your SIRT
5 a day

Super-quick to make in your favourite juicer.

Serves 1 • *Ready in 2 minutes*

¼ avocado, stoned, peeled and roughly chopped

1 kiwi, peeled, halved, seeds scraped out
with a teaspoon

100ml freshly pressed apple juice

½ ripe pear, cored, peeled and roughly chopped

30g young spinach leaves, stalks removed

1 Simply place in the juicer or blender and blend until smooth.

Summer Watermelon Juice

126 calories

1
of your SIRT
5 a day

A fresh, summery juice.

Serves 1 • Ready in 2 minutes

½ cucumber, peeled if preferred, halved,
seeds removed and roughly chopped

20g young kale leaves, stalks removed

4 mint leaves

250g watermelon chunks

1   Just whizz in your juicer or blender and enjoy immediately.

Grape and Melon Juice

125 calories

2
of your SIRT
5 a day

A little ray of sunshine in a glass.

Serves 1 • *Ready in 2 minutes*

½ cucumber, peeled if preferred, halved,
seeds removed and roughly chopped

30g young spinach leaves, stalks removed

100g red seedless grapes

100g cantaloupe melon, peeled, deseeded
and cut into chunks

1 Blend together in a juicer or blender until smooth.

SIRT Fruit Salad

172 calories

3
of your SIRT
5 a day

This fruit salad is packed full of the best fruit SIRTs.

Serves 1 • Ready in 10 minutes

½ cup freshly made green tea
1 tsp honey
1 orange, halved
1 apple, cored and roughly chopped
10 red seedless grapes
10 blueberries

1 Stir the honey into half a cup of green tea. When dissolved, add the juice of half the orange. Leave to cool.

2 Chop the other half of the orange and place in a bowl together with the chopped apple, grapes and blueberries. Pour over the cooled tea and leave to steep for a few minutes before serving.

Green Tea Smoothie

183 calories

1
of your SIRT
5 a day

This super-healthy smoothie uses matcha powder, which is a highly concentrated Japanese green tea. It can be found in specialist Asian or tea shops.

Serves 2 • Ready in 3 minutes

2 ripe bananas
250ml milk
2 tsp matcha green tea powder
½ tsp vanilla bean paste (not extract) or a small scrape of the seeds from a vanilla pod
6 ice cubes
2 tsp honey

1 Simply blend all the ingredients together in a blender and serve in two glasses.

Kale and Blackcurrant Smoothie

86 calories

1½
of your SIRT
5 a day

If you want to get all your SIRTs in one hit, then this is the smoothie to do it. It has a delicious, healthy zing.

Serves 2 • Ready in 3 minutes

2 tsp honey
1 cup freshly made green tea
10 baby kale leaves, stalks removed
1 ripe banana
40g blackcurrants, washed and stalks removed
6 ice cubes

1 Stir the honey into the warm green tea until dissolved. Whizz all the ingredients together in a blender until smooth. Serve immediately.

Blueberry Smoothie

160 calories

1
of your SIRT
5 a day

This yogurt smoothie has a rich, creamy taste.

Serves 2 • Ready in 2 minutes

1 ripe banana
100g blueberries
100g blackberries
2 tbsp natural yogurt
200ml milk

1 Blend all the ingredients together until smooth.

Blackcurrant and Oat Yogurt Swirl

241 calories

1½
of your SIRT
5 a day

The simple blackcurrant compote can be made in advance and refrigerated. This means that this delicious and filling yogurt can be ready in minutes.

Serves 2 • Ready in 10 minutes

100g blackcurrants, washed and stalks removed
2 tbsp caster sugar
100ml water
200g natural yogurt
40g jumbo oats

1 Place the blackcurrants, sugar and water in a small pan and bring to the boil. Reduce the heat slightly, keeping a vigorous simmer, and continue to cook for 5 minutes. Turn off the heat and leave to cool. The blackcurrant compote can now be refrigerated until needed.

2 Place the yogurt and oats in a large bowl and stir together. Distribute the blackcurrant compote between two serving bowls and top with the yogurt and oats. Use a cocktail stick to swirl the compote through the yogurt. Serve immediately.

Green Omelette

234 calories

2½
of your SIRT
5 a day

If you want a healthy and protein-rich start to the day, you can't go wrong with this appetising green omelette.

Serves 1 • Ready in 10 minutes

1 tsp olive oil

1 shallot, peeled and finely chopped

2 large eggs, at room temperature

Handful (20g) rocket leaves

Small handful (10g) parsley, finely chopped

Salt and freshly ground black pepper

1 In a wide frying pan, heat the oil on a medium-low heat and gently fry the shallot for 5 minutes. Turn the heat up a little bit and cook for another 2 minutes.

2 In a bowl or cup, whisk the eggs together well with a fork. Distribute the shallot evenly around the pan before pouring in the eggs. Tip the pan slightly to each side so that the egg is evenly distributed. Cook for a minute or so before lifting the sides of the omelette and letting any runny egg slip into the base of the pan. Immediately sprinkle over the rocket leaves and parsley and season generously with salt and pepper.

3 When cooked, the top of the omelette will still be soft but not runny and the base will be just starting to brown. Tip onto a plate and enjoy straight away.

Choc Chip Granola

244 calories

½
of your SIRT
5 a day

Chocolate at breakfast – don't mind if I do. Be sure to serve with a cup of green tea to give you plenty of SIRTs. The rice malt syrup can be substituted with maple syrup if you prefer.

Serves 8 • Ready in 30 minutes

200g jumbo oats
50g pecans, roughly chopped
3 tbsp light olive oil
20g butter
1 tbsp dark brown sugar
2 tbsp rice malt syrup
60g good-quality (70%) dark chocolate chips

1 Preheat the oven to 160°C (140°C fan/Gas 3). Line a large baking tray with a silicone sheet or baking parchment.

2 Mix the oats and pecans together in a large bowl. In a small non-stick pan, gently heat the olive oil, butter, brown sugar and rice malt syrup until the butter has melted and the sugar and syrup have dissolved. Do not allow to boil. Pour the syrup over the oats and stir thoroughly until the oats are fully covered.

3 Distribute the granola over the baking tray, spreading right into the corners. Leave clumps of mixture with spacing rather than an even spread. Bake in the oven for 20 minutes until just tinged golden brown at the edges. Remove from the oven and leave to cool on the tray completely.

4 When cool, break up any bigger lumps on the tray with your fingers and then mix in the chocolate chips. Scoop or pour the granola into an airtight tub or jar. The granola will keep for at least 2 weeks.

Raspberry and Blackcurrant Jelly

76 calories

2
of your SIRT
5 a day

Making a jelly in advance is a great way to prepare the fruit so that it is ready to eat first thing in the morning.

Serves 2 • Ready in 15 minutes + setting time

100g raspberries, washed
2 leaves gelatine
100g blackcurrants, washed and stalks removed
2 tbsp granulated sugar
300ml water

1 Arrange the raspberries in two serving dishes/glasses/moulds. Put the gelatine leaves in a bowl of cold water to soften.

2 Place the blackcurrants in a small pan with the sugar and 100ml water and bring to the boil. Simmer vigorously for 5 minutes and then remove from the heat. Leave to stand for 2 minutes.

3 Squeeze out excess water from the gelatine leaves and add them to the saucepan. Stir until fully dissolved, then stir in the rest of the water. Pour the liquid into the prepared dishes and refrigerate to set. The jellies should be ready in about 3–4 hours or overnight.

Apple Pancakes with Blackcurrant Compote

337 calories

1½
of your SIRT
5 a day

These pancakes are decadent but healthy. A great lazy morning treat.

Serves 4 • Ready in 20 minutes

75g porridge oats
125g plain flour
1 tsp baking powder
2 tbsp caster sugar
Pinch of salt
2 apples, peeled, cored and cut into small pieces
300ml semi-skimmed milk
2 egg whites
2 tsp light olive oil

For the compote:

120g blackcurrants, washed and stalks removed
2 tbsp caster sugar
3 tbsp water

1 First make the compote. Place the blackcurrants, sugar and water in a small pan. Bring up to a simmer and cook for 10–15 minutes.

2 Place the oats, flour, baking powder, caster sugar and salt in a large bowl and mix well. Stir in the apple and then whisk in the milk a little at a time until you have a smooth mixture. Whisk the egg whites to stiff peaks and then fold into the pancake batter. Transfer the batter to a jug.

3 Heat ½ tsp oil in a non-stick frying pan on a medium-high heat and pour in approximately one quarter of the batter. Cook on both sides until golden brown. Remove and repeat to make four pancakes.

4 Serve the pancakes with the blackcurrant compote drizzled over.

SIMPLE SNACKS

Simple, unusual and healthy snacks.

• • •

Peanut Energy Bars

Turmeric Roasted Nuts

Crunchy Kale Seaweed

Wasabi Peas

Fried Chilli Tofu

Olive Tapenade

Crunchy Fried Olives

Turmeric Apple Chips

Chocolate Shots

Frozen Chocolate Grapes

Chocolate Matcha Energy Balls

Peanut Energy Bars

135 calories

⅓
of your SIRT
5 a day

I love these filling, tasty and low-sugar energy bars. I make them all the time for myself and the kids and they always get eaten superfast. You can wrap the bars individually in clingfilm to make a great on-the-go or lunchbox snack. Peanuts, lemon, olive oil and dark chocolate are all SIRT foods.

Serves 16 • Ready in 35 minutes + setting time

50g blanched (unsalted) peanuts
200g jumbo oats
Zest of 1 lemon (washed in hot soapy water to remove wax first)
50ml light olive oil
30g butter
25g dark brown sugar
2 heaped tbsp (50g) rice malt syrup
Juice of ½ lemon
50g good-quality (70%) dark chocolate chips

1 Lightly grease a 15cm square cake tin. Preheat the oven to 160°C (140°C fan/Gas 3).

2 In a large bowl, combine the peanuts, oats and lemon zest. ☛

3 To a small non-stick pan, add the olive oil, butter, brown sugar, rice malt syrup and lemon juice. Heat gently, stirring all the time until the butter has melted and the ingredients have combined.

4 Remove from the heat and pour over the peanut/oat mixture. Keep stirring until the oats are fully coated. Scoop out the mix into the prepared cake tin. Level out with the back of the spoon, pressing down firmly as you go.

5 Bake for 20 minutes until just tinged golden at the edges. Remove from the oven but leave in the tin.

6 While the energy bars are still hot, sprinkle the chocolate chips over and leave to melt for about 10 minutes. Use a knife to spread the dark chocolate evenly over the bars and leave to cool – still in the tin – until the chocolate has set.

7 Carefully remove the whole cake from the tin and place on a chopping board. With a very sharp knife cut into 16 squares. When fully cool, store in an airtight container for up to 5 days.

Turmeric Roasted Nuts

195 calories

½
of your SIRT
5 a day

Peanuts are a surprising source of SIRTs and can be combined with turmeric to make this very moreish snack.

Serves 8 • Ready in 25 minutes

250g blanched peanuts
1 tbsp honey
1 tbsp granulated sugar
1 tsp ground cumin
1 tsp salt
½ tsp chilli powder
½ tsp ground turmeric
½ tsp smoked paprika

1 Preheat the oven to 160°C (140°C fan/Gas 3). Line a baking tray with a silicone sheet or baking parchment.

2 In a large bowl, mix the peanuts with the honey. In a separate small bowl, combine the sugar, cumin, salt, chilli powder, turmeric and smoked paprika. Add the sugar and spice mix to the peanuts and toss well to coat evenly. Spread the peanuts onto the prepared baking tray.

3 Bake for approximately 20 minutes, stirring every 5 minutes, until the coating has started to thicken. Remove from the oven and leave to cool completely on the tray. ☞

4 Break up any large lumps and store in an airtight container for up to 2 weeks.

Crunchy Kale Seaweed

81 calories

2
of your SIRT
5 a day

An amazing tasty and easy snack made from one of the richest SIRT sources.

Serves 2 • Ready in 12 minutes

100g kale, washed

1 tbsp extra virgin olive oil

Freshly ground sea salt and black pepper

1 Preheat the oven to 200°C (180°C fan/Gas 6).

2 Remove the chewy stalks from the kale and roughly chop. Dry the kale on kitchen paper if necessary and place on a large baking tray.

3 Drizzle with the olive oil and sprinkle on a generous quantity of sea salt and a little black pepper.

4 Cook in the oven for 8–10 minutes. Remove from the oven and allow to cool completely on the tray. Best served the same day.

Wasabi Peas

98 calories

1
of your SIRT
5 a day

I am a little bit addicted to these ... The edamame and wasabi powder both contain the all-important SIRTs, so feel free to indulge.

Serves 4 • Ready in 35 minutes + drying time

250g fresh or frozen soya/edamame beans
6 tsp wasabi powder
1 tsp salt
¼ tsp onion powder
4 tsp water

1 If you have frozen soya beans, then you can defrost fully on kitchen paper and pat dry.
2 Preheat the oven to 160°C (140°C fan/Gas 3). Dry the soya beans with kitchen paper before spreading out on a baking tray and cooking for 30 minutes.
3 Five minutes before the end of the cooking time, place the wasabi powder, salt and onion powder in a bowl and whisk together with the water to make a smooth paste. Cover and leave to rest for 5 minutes.
4 When the beans have cooked, remove from the oven and immediately scoop into the wasabi paste. Stir thoroughly so that all surfaces of the beans are coated and pour back

into the baking tray to cool and dry out. Leave in the baking tray for about an hour before transferring to an airtight container.

Fried Chilli Tofu

132 calories

This makes a quick and easy lunch or snack.

Serves 1 • Ready in 15 minutes

150g firm tofu, cut into cubes
1 clove garlic, peeled and crushed
Juice of ½ lemon
½ tsp chilli flakes
½ tsp paprika
½ tsp ground turmeric
Salt and freshly ground black pepper
1 tsp oil

1 Spread the tofu out on a plate covered in kitchen paper. Cover with kitchen paper and set aside to dry out.

2 Place the garlic, lemon juice, spices and a generous seasoning of salt and pepper in a wide bowl. Mix together before adding the tofu and gently tossing through so that

the tofu is fully covered. Leave to stand for between 5 and 15 minutes.

3 Heat the oil in a frying pan on a medium-high heat and wait until the pan is hot before removing the tofu from the marinade and adding to the pan. Fry for 3–4 minutes, stirring every minute or so, until the tofu is golden brown all over. Turn off the heat, then add the remaining marinade to the pan and serve.

Olive Tapenade

132 calories

2
of your SIRT
5 a day

Tapenade is stuffed full of SIRTs – olives, anchovies, capers, olive oil – so use as a versatile topping to meats or just as a dip with pitta or vegetables. You can use green or black olives in this recipe to get slightly different flavours, just make sure you get pitted olives in oil.

Serves 4 • *Ready in 5 minutes*

1 clove garlic, peeled and crushed

Zest and juice of ½ lemon (washed in hot soapy water to remove wax first)

1 tbsp capers, drained

3 anchovy fillets, drained and roughly chopped

☞

200g pitted green or black olives, drained

2 tbsp extra virgin olive oil

1 Place the garlic, lemon zest and juice, capers and anchovies in a food processor and blend until smooth. Add the olives and blend again. Don't over-blend as a few olive pieces make for a more interesting texture.

2 Scoop out the paste and stir through the olive oil. The tapenade will keep for a few days in the fridge. As with all olives, it will taste better served at room temperature.

Crunchy Fried Olives

343 calories

2½
of your SIRT
5 a day

An absolutely beautiful way to serve olives.

Serves 2 • Ready in 5 minutes

200g green pitted olives

1 egg, beaten

50g panko breadcrumbs

½ tsp ground turmeric

½ tsp paprika

1 tbsp olive oil

1 Dry the olives on kitchen paper. Place the beaten eggs in one shallow bowl and mix the breadcrumbs, turmeric and paprika in another.

2 Dip and coat the olives first in the beaten egg and then roll in the breadcrumbs.

3 Heat the oil in a wide frying pan on a medium heat. When hot, add the coated olives and fry until golden brown all over. Remove with a slotted spoon and drain on kitchen paper before serving.

Turmeric Apple Chips

58 calories

1
of your SIRT
5 a day

These scrumptious little treats will keep in an airtight container for several days.

Serves 1 • Ready in 1½ hours

Juice of ½ lemon
¼ tsp ground turmeric
½ tsp ground cinnamon
½ tsp ground ginger
1 large eating apple

1 Preheat the oven to 120°C (100°C fan/Gas ½). Line two baking sheets with baking parchment or silicone sheets. ☞

2   Place the lemon juice in a small bowl and mix in the spices. Cut off the top of the apple. Use a peeler to cut very thin circles of apple across the top. Any seeds in the centre will just fall out. As each very thin slice is peeled off, drop it into the lemon juice and lightly toss a little lemon juice over the top to prevent browning. Discard the base of the apple.

3   Arrange the apple rings in a single layer over the baking sheets. Bake for 1 hour 15 minutes, turning after 45 minutes. Remove from the oven and allow to cool and crisp on the baking tray before storing in an airtight container.

Chocolate Shots

68 calories

1
of your SIRT
5 a day

Best used when you have a chocolate craving to satisfy. Use the zaniest shot glasses you can for extra effect.

Serves 2 • Ready in 1 minute

2 heaped tsp (20g) good-quality cocoa powder

2 tsp (10g) granulated sugar

A little boiling water

60ml milk

1   Place the cocoa and sugar in a small jug. Add a little water from the kettle, just enough to make a smooth paste.

Pour in the milk a little at a time, stirring thoroughly. Pour into two shot glasses and enjoy your chocolate hit immediately.

Frozen Chocolate Grapes

97 calories

1
of your SIRT
5 a day

These are a great healthy snack to have in your freezer. Serve in an olive dish with a cocktail stick for added class.

Serves 4 • Ready in 10 minutes + freezing time

50g good-quality (70%) dark chocolate

150g red seedless grapes

1 Line a baking tray with a silicone sheet or baking parchment.
2 Break up the chocolate into small pieces and place in a small heatproof bowl. Heat a small pan of water to a gentle simmer and place the bowl containing the chocolate on top. Make sure the bowl does not touch the water.
3 Heat and stir the chocolate so that it melts slowly and remove from the heat when it still has a few lumps remaining. Continue to stir the chocolate until it is all melted (this helps to prevent white patches or blooming on the chocolate). ☞

4 Dip the grapes into the chocolate one at a time, so that they are half coated, and place immediately on the baking tray. Continue with all the grapes.

5 Leave the chocolate to set at room temperature before transferring to the freezer. Once frozen the grapes can be moved to a suitable freezer container.

6 Serve in portions of 10 to 12 grapes at a time or just reach in and grab a few when the need arises.

Chocolate Matcha Energy Balls

111 calories

1
of your SIRT
5 a day

These balls give you a fabulous burst of energy.

Makes 10 balls • Ready in 10 minutes

100g soft pitted dates
100g blanched almonds
50g good-quality cocoa powder
1 tbsp matcha green tea powder + more for dusting
2 tbsp almond milk

1 Place the dates and almonds in a food processor and process until they come together into a sticky ball. Break up the ball with a fork and add the cocoa, matcha and almond milk. Blend until they form a large sticky ball.

2 Scoop out large heaped teaspoons of the mix and roll into small tight balls. Repeat until you have 10 to 12 balls. Dust over a little more matcha powder. These balls will keep refrigerated for up to 2 weeks.

QUICK FIXES

No time to cook? These light meals can be
whipped up in minutes. Lunchboxes are a
perfect choice for a work day.

● ● ●

Spicy Bean Burgers with Spinach Salad

Greek Salad Skewers

Egg Florentine

Roast Chicken and Pesto Wrap

No-Cook Falafel Lunchbox

Mexican Salsa with Wensleydale and
Cucumber Pittas

Brie and Grape Salad Lunchbox

Herby Chicken Lunchbox

Spicy Bean Burgers with Spinach Salad

230 calories

4
of your SIRT
5 a day

Delicious and so quick to prepare. Extras can be saved and eaten hot or cold the next day.

Serves 2 • Ready in 10 minutes

1 × 400g tin cannellini beans, rinsed and drained

1 tbsp tomato purée

1 tbsp cornflour

2 spring onions, trimmed and chopped

1 clove garlic, peeled and crushed

1 tsp chilli flakes

½ tsp ground turmeric

Handful (10g) flat-leaf parsley, finely chopped

Salt and freshly ground black pepper

1 tbsp olive oil

For the salad:

100g baby spinach leaves

50g cucumber, halved lengthways and sliced

2 tsp extra virgin olive oil

2 tsp lemon juice

1 Place the beans in a large bowl and use a potato masher or fork to thoroughly mash the beans. Add the tomato purée, cornflour, spring onion, garlic, chilli flakes, turmeric and parsley. Season generously with salt and pepper. Mix well.

2 Divide the mixture into four portions and form into balls, then flatten a little to form a burger. If you have time, chill for 20 minutes or keep refrigerated until needed. The burgers will hold their shape slightly better if chilled but will be just as delicious if cooked straight away.

3 Heat the oil in a wide frying pan over a medium heat. Add the burgers to the pan and cook for 3–4 minutes. Turn with a fish slice and flatten a little more if necessary. Cook for a further 3–4 minutes until golden brown.

4 Prepare the salad over two serving plates. Distribute the spinach and cucumber over both plates. Drizzle the olive oil and lemon juice over. Serve with two burgers arranged over the top and an extra squeeze of lemon.

Greek Salad Skewers

306 calories

3½
of your SIRT
5 a day

These colourful sticks of goodness look so cheery. They taste of summer.

Serves 2 • Ready in 10 minutes

2 wooden skewers, soaked in water for
30 minutes before use

8 large black olives

8 cherry tomatoes

1 yellow pepper, cut into 8 squares

½ red onion, cut in half and separated into 8 pieces

100g (about 10cm) cucumber, cut into 4 slices and halved

100g feta, cut into 8 cubes

For the dressing:

1 tbsp extra virgin olive oil

Juice of ½ lemon

1 tsp balsamic vinegar

½ clove garlic, peeled and crushed

Few leaves basil, finely chopped (or ½ tsp dried
mixed herbs to replace basil and oregano)

Few leaves oregano, finely chopped

Generous seasoning of salt and freshly ground black pepper

☛

1 Thread each skewer with the salad ingredients in the order: olive, tomato, yellow pepper, red onion, cucumber, feta, tomato, olive, yellow pepper, red onion, cucumber, feta.

2 Place all the dressing ingredients in a small bowl and mix together thoroughly. Pour over the skewers.

Egg Florentine

215 calories

2
of your SIRT
5 a day

A lovely quick meal for one.

Serves 1 • Ready in 10 minutes

1 large egg
1 tbsp thick mayonnaise
¼ tsp Dijon mustard
Juice of ½ lemon
1 tsp extra virgin olive oil
Pinch of salt
¼ tsp ground turmeric
¼ tsp cayenne pepper
1 tsp capers
1 tsp (5g) butter
¼ tsp nutmeg

50g fresh spinach, stalks removed

Pinch of paprika

1 Fill a shallow saucepan with 4–5cm water. Bring to a gentle simmer. Crack the egg on the side of the pan and lower slowly into the water. Simmer for exactly 1 minute. Turn off the heat and leave to cook in the slowly cooling water for a further 9 minutes. This should ensure a cooked egg with a runny middle.

2 Next prepare the mock hollandaise. Mix the mayonnaise, mustard, lemon juice, olive oil, salt, turmeric and cayenne in a small bowl until smooth. Stir in the capers.

3 In a small lidded pan, heat the butter and nutmeg until the butter is just starting to sizzle. Add the spinach and stir through for 30 seconds. Then place the lid on the pan, turn off the heat and allow the spinach to wilt for 2 minutes.

4 To serve, place the wilted spinach on a small plate, use a slotted spoon to remove the egg carefully from the water and place on top of the spinach. Pour over the hollandaise sauce and top with a pinch of paprika.

Roast Chicken and Pesto Wrap

404 calories

2
of your SIRT
5 a day

This makes enough pesto for four wraps. If you make up the pesto in advance, then the wrap can be very quickly made for a healthy alternative to a sandwich.

Serves 4 • Ready in 8 minutes

For the pesto:

50g rocket leaves

30g basil leaves

½ clove garlic, peeled and chopped

½ tsp sea salt

50g pine nuts

20g Parmesan cheese, finely grated

2 tbsp extra virgin olive oil

Good squeeze of lemon juice

For each wrap:

1 soft tortilla wrap

Handful baby spinach leaves

1 small roasted chicken breast fillet (100g), sliced

1 Place the rocket, basil, garlic and sea salt into a food processor and pulse until roughly chopped. Add the pine nuts and Parmesan and pulse again, leaving the pine nuts relatively coarse. Stir in the olive oil and lemon juice. Transfer to a suitable container and leave for the flavours to develop.

2 To make the wrap, arrange the spinach leaves over the central third of the tortilla wrap. Add the chicken and pour over the pesto. Then turn up the bottom 2cm of the wrap, tuck one edge firmly over the filling and then roll the rest of the wrap around as snugly as you dare. Wrap firmly in clingfilm and chill until needed.

No-Cook Falafel Lunchbox

387 calories

4
of your SIRT
5 a day

Make up a week's worth of healthy SIRT-rich lunches. Each part of the lunchbox – the falafel, tahini sauce and parsley salad – can be made in advance and will keep for several days in the fridge. When you want to serve, just place the salad in a serving dish or container, add the falafel and drizzle on the tahini sauce. If it's a portable lunchbox you need, just store one portion of tahini sauce in a small lidded container and pour over just before eating.

Serves 4 • *Ready in 45 minutes*

For the falafel:

80g unsalted shelled pistachios

30g sesame seeds

¼ tsp ground cumin

¼ tsp ground coriander

¼ tsp ground turmeric

½ clove garlic, peeled and sliced

30g flat-leaf parsley

Salt and freshly ground black pepper

For the tahini sauce:

2 tbsp (30g) tahini

1 tbsp white wine vinegar

Juice of ½ lemon

2 tbsp extra virgin olive oil

½ clove garlic, peeled

30g flat-leaf parsley, roughly chopped

Pinch of salt

For the parsley salad:

150g couscous

Juice of 2 lemons

1 tbsp extra virgin olive oil

Salt and freshly ground black pepper

¼ tsp ground cinnamon

¼ tsp ground coriander

Pinch of ground cloves

Pinch of ground ginger

4 tomatoes, finely chopped

2 spring onions, finely sliced

50g flat-leaf parsley, stalks discarded,
leaves very finely chopped

1 To make the falafel balls, simply pulse all the ingredients in a food processor until you have coarse breadcrumbs. Remove heaped teaspoons from the food processor and form into balls by rolling in your hands. Set aside or refrigerate in a lidded container until needed.

2 To make the tahini sauce, place all the ingredients in a blender and blend until smooth. Add a little water to thin if necessary. Set aside or refrigerate in a lidded container until needed.

3 To make the parsley salad, place the couscous in a bowl and add the lemon juice, extra virgin olive oil and plenty of salt and pepper. Add all the spices, erring on the side of caution especially with the cinnamon and cloves. Stir to combine. Pour over enough water so that the couscous is generously covered. Leave to rest for approximately 10 minutes until all the water is absorbed and the couscous has swelled and is cooked 'al dente'. Keep topping up the water when required during the rest period. Meanwhile combine the tomato, spring onion and parsley. Mix the salad into the spicy couscous and allow the flavours to meld for at least 5 minutes before serving.

Mexican Salsa with Wensleydale and Cucumber Pittas

324 calories

1½
of your SIRT
5 a day

This salsa tastes better and better the more you leave it and makes a great lunchbox filler.

Serves 4 • Ready in 10 minutes

¼ red onion, roughly chopped
1 small green chilli, trimmed and deseeded (leave the seeds in if you like it hot)
1 spring onion, trimmed and roughly chopped
1 clove garlic, peeled
4 large tomatoes, roughly chopped
30g flat-leaf parsley
½ tsp salt
1 tsp olive oil
Juice of 1 lime
1 tsp tomato purée
1 tbsp water

For each person:

30g Wensleydale cheese, grated
50g (5cm) cucumber, chopped
1 wholemeal pitta, quartered

1 Place the red onion, chilli, spring onion and garlic in a food processor and whizz until finely chopped. Add the tomatoes, parsley, salt, olive oil, lime juice, tomato purée and water. Pulse until just chopped. Transfer to a bowl and leave for as long as possible for the flavours to infuse.

2 Mix the Wensleydale and cucumber together and divide among the pittas. Drizzle the salsa over or dip if you prefer.

Brie and Grape Salad Lunchbox

378 calories

4
of your SIRT
5 a day

The salad and dressing can be made up separately and then combined at lunchtime. A small pot with a secure lid is perfect for the dressing.

Serves 1 • Ready in 5 minutes

50g baby kale
50g (5cm) cucumber, halved lengthways and sliced
Small handful (10g) flat-leaf parsley, leaves only
30g Brie, cut into chunks
About 10 red seedless grapes, halved
20g walnuts, halved

For the dressing:

1 tsp sesame oil
1 tsp extra virgin olive oil
Juice of ½ lime
½ tsp brown sugar
½ tsp salt

1 Simply place the kale, cucumber and parsley on a serving plate or in a lunchbox. Arrange the Brie, grapes and walnuts over the top.

2 Place all the dressing ingredients in a small dish (or lidded pot) and mix together. When you are ready to serve the salad, pour the dressing over.

Herby Chicken Lunchbox

272 calories

4
of your SIRT
5 a day

Make the dressing in a small lidded container and drizzle over the salad at lunchtime.

Serves 1 • Ready in 5 minutes

50g fresh or frozen soya/edamame beans
50g watercress leaves
Small handful (10g) flat-leaf parsley, leaves only

¼ red onion, cut into very thin slices

1 small roasted chicken breast fillet (100g), sliced

For the dressing:

2 tsp extra virgin olive oil

Juice of ½ lemon

Pinch of sugar

2 leaves parsley, finely chopped

2 leaves basil, finely chopped

2 leaves mint, finely chopped

Salt and freshly ground black pepper

1 If the soya beans are frozen or require cooking, cook as per the packet instructions and leave to cool.

2 Arrange the watercress, edamame, parsley and red onion in a serving dish or lunchbox container. Add the chicken.

3 Mix together the olive oil, lemon juice, sugar, parsley, basil and mint in a small bowl or container. Season generously with salt and pepper. Drizzle over the salad just before serving.

SUPER SALADS

These simple salads are easy to make for one or two people. If the salad is just for you, make it up one day and have the second portion the next day.

• • •

French Country Salad

Garlic Butter Chicken with Rocket Salad

Edamame Salad with Grilled Tofu

Baked Salmon Salad with Creamy Mint Dressing

Pomegranate, Feta and Walnut Salad

Serrano Ham Salad

Smoked Salmon and New Potato Salad

Salad Niçoise

Sesame Chicken Salad

LA Green Salad

Hot Chipolata and Redcurrant Salad

Brie and Grape Salad with Honey Dressing

Roast Chicken and Kale Salad with Peanut Dressing

Smoked Trout Salad

French Country Salad

245 calories

5
of your SIRT
5 a day

The addition of the cannellini beans makes this a filling and hearty salad. The rest times are important to develop the best flavour of the salad.

Serves 2 • Ready in 15 minutes

1 sprig mint (5g), finely chopped
1 sprig basil (5g), finely chopped
1 tbsp extra virgin olive oil
Juice of 1 lemon
1 tsp Dijon mustard
Pinch of sugar
Salt and freshly ground black pepper
1 × 400g tin cannellini beans, rinsed and drained
1 red onion, chopped
1 large handful (20g) parsley, finely chopped
4 tomatoes, roughly chopped
½ cucumber, roughly cubed

1 Place the chopped mint, basil, olive oil, lemon juice, mustard and sugar in a small bowl. Add a generous seasoning of salt and pepper. Leave to rest for 5 minutes. ☞

2 Place the cannellini beans, red onion, parsley, tomatoes and cucumber in a larger bowl. Pour over the dressing and stir to incorporate. Leave to rest for 5 minutes before serving.

Garlic Butter Chicken with Rocket Salad

334 calories

3
of your SIRT
5 a day

A very flavoursome chicken salad.

Serves 2 • *Ready in 15 minutes*

2 cloves garlic, peeled and crushed
1 tbsp extra virgin olive oil
½ tsp dried oregano/mixed herbs
Freshly ground black pepper
20g butter, at room temperature
2 × 150g skinless chicken breast fillets, cut into strips
80g rocket leaves
½ red onion, cut into very thin strips
Large handful (20g) parsley, roughly chopped
½ cucumber, halved lengthways, deseeded with a teaspoon and sliced
1 tsp white wine vinegar

1 In a small bowl, combine the garlic, olive oil, dried herbs and black pepper. Set aside 1 teaspoon of the mixture to dress the salad. Add the butter to the bowl and mix until you have a smooth paste.

2 Add the garlic butter to the chicken strips and use your hands to rub the butter all over the chicken pieces.

3 Head a wide frying pan to a medium heat and when hot toss in the chicken strips. Cook for 10–14 minutes until browned and fully cooked, stirring regularly. Remove from the pan. The chicken can be used hot or cold in the salad.

4 Arrange the rocket, red onion, parsley and cucumber over two serving plates. Add the white wine vinegar to the set aside garlic oil and pour over the two salads. Top with the cooked chicken.

Edamame Salad with Grilled Tofu

293 calories

3
of your SIRT
5 a day

This is an unusual and very healthy salad.

Serves 2 • Ready in 15 minutes

200g firm tofu, thickly sliced

150g fresh or frozen soya/edamame beans

1 shallot, peeled and very thinly sliced

100g beansprouts
½ cucumber, halved lengthways, deseeded with a teaspoon and sliced
Large handful (20g) flat-leaf parsley, roughly chopped
1 tsp sesame oil
Salt and freshly ground black pepper

For the dressing:

2 tbsp mirin
2 tsp dark soy sauce
Zest and juice of ½ orange (washed in hot soapy water to remove wax first)
½ tsp chilli flakes

1 Spread the tofu out on a plate covered in kitchen paper. Cover with kitchen paper and set aside to dry out.

2 If the soya beans are frozen or require cooking, cook as per the packet instructions and leave to cool.

3 Mix the edamame, shallot, beansprouts, cucumber and parsley together in a bowl. Combine all the dressing ingredients and pour over the salad. Stir gently to combine.

4 Heat the grill or griddle to a high temperature. Brush the tofu with the sesame oil on both sides, season generously with salt and pepper and place on the grill tray or griddle. Cook for 2–3 minutes each side, turning carefully with a fish slice.

5 Divide the salad between two serving plates and arrange the tofu over the top.

Baked Salmon Salad with Creamy Mint Dressing

340 calories

3
of your SIRT
5 a day

Baking the salmon in the oven makes this salad so simple.

Serves 1 • Ready in 20 minutes

1 salmon fillet (130g)
40g mixed salad leaves
40g young spinach leaves
2 radishes, trimmed and thinly sliced
5cm piece (50g) cucumber, cut into chunks
2 spring onions, trimmed and sliced
1 small handful (10g) parsley, roughly chopped

For the dressing:

1 tsp low-fat mayonnaise
1 tbsp natural yogurt
1 tbsp rice vinegar
2 leaves mint, finely chopped
Salt and freshly ground black pepper

1 Preheat the oven to 200°C (180°C fan/Gas 6).
2 Place the salmon fillet on a baking tray and bake for 16–18 minutes until just cooked through. Remove from the

oven and set aside. The salmon is equally nice hot or cold in the salad. If your salmon has skin, simply cook skin side down and remove the salmon from the skin using a fish slice after cooking. It should slide off easily when cooked.

3 In a small bowl, mix together the mayonnaise, yogurt, rice wine vinegar, mint leaves and salt and pepper together and leave to stand for at least 5 minutes to allow the flavours to develop.

4 Arrange the salad leaves and spinach on a serving plate and top with the radishes, cucumber, spring onions and parsley. Flake the cooked salmon onto the salad and drizzle the dressing over.

Pomegranate, Feta and Walnut Salad

390 calories

1½
of your SIRT
5 a day

A totally delicious combination of flavours.

Serves 1 • *Ready in 5 minutes*

75g young spinach leaves, roughly chopped

50g ready-to-eat or cooked puy lentils

30g feta cheese, cut into cubes

20g pomegranate seeds

20g walnuts, halved

For the dressing:

1 tbsp Greek-style yogurt
1 tsp rice vinegar
Pinch of sugar
1 tsp olive oil
2 leaves mint, finely chopped

1 Combine all the dressing ingredients in a small bowl.
2 Arrange the spinach leaves and lentils on a serving dish. Top with the feta, pomegranate and walnuts. Drizzle the dressing over the top and serve.

Serrano Ham Salad

298 calories

5
of your SIRT
5 a day

This serrano ham salad combines the most SIRT-rich ingredients possible. The sweetness of the blackcurrants beautifully offsets the saltiness of the ham and olives.

Serves 1 • Ready in 5 minutes

40g baby kale
40g young spinach leaves
Small handful (10g) parsley, stalks discarded and roughly chopped

2 slices (30g) serrano ham, chopped

About 12 pitted Kalamata olives, halved

Handful (30g) blackcurrants, washed
and stalks removed

For the dressing:

1 tsp capers, drained

1 tsp extra virgin olive oil

Juice of ½ lemon

Salt and freshly ground black pepper

1 Combine the capers, olive oil, lemon juice and salt and pepper in a small bowl and set aside.

2 Mix the kale, spinach and parsley lightly in a serving dish. Arrange the serrano ham, olives and blackcurrants over the top. Pour over the dressing and serve immediately.

Smoked Salmon and New Potato Salad

348 calories

4
of your SIRT
5 a day

Filling, easy and one of my favourites.

Serves 1 • Ready in 25 minutes

120g new potatoes, quartered

50g frozen soya/edamame beans

80g young spinach leaves

40g smoked salmon, cut into strips

For the dressing:

2 tsp extra virgin olive oil

1 shallot, peeled and very finely chopped

1 tsp balsamic vinegar

½ tsp English mustard

Salt and freshly ground black pepper

1 Steam the new potatoes for 18–20 minutes until tender. Add the soya beans for the last 4 minutes of the cooking time. Set aside to cool.

2 Heat the extra virgin olive oil very gently in a small pan. Add the shallot and fry lightly for 5 minutes. Remove from the heat and add the balsamic vinegar, mustard and salt and pepper.

3 Arrange the spinach leaves over a serving plate. Add the new potatoes and edamame beans. Lightly toss through the dressing. Finally, arrange the smoked salmon over the top.

Salad Niçoise

456 calories

3
of your SIRT
5 a day

You can't beat a traditional ... ish Salad Niçoise.

Serves 2 • Ready in 40 minutes

250g new potatoes, quartered

50g fresh or frozen soya/edamame beans

2 large eggs

4 large tomatoes, roughly chopped

10cm piece (150g) cucumber, halved
lengthways and sliced

½ red pepper, thinly sliced

50g good-quality black olives, pitted

1 tbsp capers, rinsed and drained

4 anchovy fillets, cut into thin slices

Large handful (20g) parsley, roughly chopped

For the dressing:

1 clove garlic, peeled

2 anchovies, roughly chopped

3–4 basil leaves

Salt and freshly ground black pepper

2 tbsp extra virgin olive oil

1 tsp red wine vinegar

1 Steam the new potatoes for 15–20 minutes until just tender. Adding the soya beans for the last 4 minutes if frozen, or the last minute if fresh. Leave to cool.

2 Prick the eggs and lower into a pan of boiling water. Boil for 9 minutes. Remove and place in a pan of cold water for a few minutes before peeling and quartering.

3 To make the dressing, use a food processor, coffee grinder or pestle and mortar to grind together the garlic, anchovies, basil leaves and salt and pepper. Stir in the olive oil and vinegar.

4 Put the tomato, cucumber, red pepper, olives, capers, anchovies and parsley in a large bowl with the potatoes and soya beans. Mix lightly to combine, add the dressing then mix again. Arrange the quartered eggs over the top just before serving.

Sesame Chicken Salad

465 calories

4
of your SIRT
5 a day

An unusual salad but very addictive.

Serves 2   •   Ready in 12 minutes

1 tbsp sesame seeds
1 cucumber, peeled, halved lengthways, deseeded with a teaspoon and sliced

☞

100g baby kale, roughly chopped

60g pak choi, very finely shredded

½ red onion, very finely sliced

Large handful (20g) parsley, chopped

150g cooked chicken, shredded

For the dressing:

1 tbsp extra virgin olive oil

1 tsp sesame oil

Juice of 1 lime

1 tsp clear honey

2 tsp soy sauce

1 Toast the sesame seeds in a dry frying pan for 2 minutes until lightly browned and fragrant. Transfer to a plate to cool.

2 In a small bowl, mix together the olive oil, sesame oil, lime juice, honey and soy sauce to make the dressing.

3 Place the cucumber, kale, pak choi, red onion and parsley in a large bowl and gently mix together. Pour over the dressing and mix again.

4 Distribute the salad between two plates and top with the shredded chicken. Sprinkle over the sesame seeds just before serving.

LA Green Salad

304 calories

2½
of your SIRT
5 a day

You can't get much healthier than an LA salad.

Serves 2 • *Ready in 15 minutes*

100g small broccoli florets
100g asparagus, trimmed
50g watercress leaves
50g spinach leaves
200g ready-to-eat or cooked puy lentils
½ ripe avocado, stoned, peeled and cut into large chunks
20g pomegranate seeds

For the dressing:

2 tsp extra virgin olive oil
¼ tsp ground cumin
¼ tsp ground turmeric
Zest and juice of 1 lemon (washed in hot soapy water to remove wax first)
2 tbsp natural yogurt

1 Steam the broccoli over a pan of boiling water for 5 minutes or until just tender. Add the asparagus for the last 2–4 minutes (2 minutes for 'al dente'). Leave to cool. ☛

2 Make the dressing by combining the olive oil, cumin, turmeric, lemon zest and juice with the natural yogurt in a small bowl.

3 Toss together the watercress and spinach leaves with the broccoli, asparagus, lentils and avocado. Add the dressing and combine gently. Divide between two serving plates and serve with the pomegranate seeds sprinkled over.

Hot Chipolata and Redcurrant Salad

309 calories

3
of your SIRT
5 a day

The sweet (and SIRT-rich) redcurrants go brilliantly well with the salty chipolatas. Freezing and then defrosting the redcurrants may seem counterintuitive, but it helps break down the skins.

Serves 2 • Ready in 25 minutes

100g small broccoli florets

1 small shallot, peeled and finely chopped

200g chipolata sausages, snipped into 2cm pieces

100g redcurrants, frozen and then fully defrosted

100g watercress

100g young spinach leaves

For the dressing:

1 tbsp olive oil
½ tsp English mustard
1 tsp clear honey
1 tsp cider vinegar
Salt and freshly ground black pepper

1 Steam the broccoli over a pan of boiling water for 5–6 minutes, then set aside to cool.

2 Heat a frying pan on a medium heat and add the shallot and chipolatas. Cook for 15–20 minutes, stirring regularly, until the chipolatas are cooked through. Turn off the heat and add the redcurrants. Stir well and leave to rest in the pan for 5 minutes.

3 Make the dressing by combining the olive oil, mustard, honey, vinegar and salt and pepper in a small bowl.

4 Put the broccoli, watercress and spinach leaves in a large bowl. Stir through half the dressing. Arrange the salad over two plates, distribute the chipolatas and redcurrants evenly between the dishes and drizzle over the last of the dressing.

Brie and Grape Salad with Honey Dressing

476 calories

3
of your SIRT
5 a day

In my opinion, grapes are totally underrated as a salad ingredient. They go particularly well with salty foods like cheese.

Serves 1 • Ready in 5 minutes

1 little gem lettuce, roughly chopped

30g rocket

½ cucumber, peeled, halved lengthways and sliced

100g red seedless grapes, halved

1 tsp capers, drained

50g Brie, cut into large chunks

20g walnuts, halved

For the dressing:

1 tsp runny honey

2 tsp red wine vinegar

2 tsp extra virgin olive oil

Pinch of salt

1 Put the lettuce, rocket leaves, cucumber, grapes and capers in a bowl and mix lightly.
2 Combine all the dressing ingredients in a small bowl and

then pour over the green salad. Arrange the Brie and walnuts over the top and simply serve.

Roast Chicken and Kale Salad with Peanut Dressing

383 calories

2
of your SIRT
5 a day

I think I might be addicted to the peanut dressing.

Serves 2 • Ready in 15 minutes

60g small broccoli florets
150g cooked and cooled basmati rice
60g baby kale, chopped
60g young spinach leaves, chopped
Small handful (10g) parsley, roughly chopped
200g cooked chicken breast, sliced
10g sesame seeds

For the dressing:

1 heaped tsp smooth peanut butter
10g creamed coconut dissolved in 30ml boiling water
Juice of ½ lime
½ tsp brown sugar
½ tsp sesame oil

1 Steam the broccoli over a pan of boiling water for 5 minutes or until just tender.

2 Put the rice in a large bowl and break up any clumps with a fork. Add the kale, spinach, broccoli and parsley and stir gently.

3 Add the dissolved coconut to the peanut butter a little bit at a time. Stir each time to ensure a smooth consistency. Add the lime juice, brown sugar and sesame oil. Divide the dressing in half and pour one half over the rice and greens and stir. Pour the rest of the dressing over the cooked chicken and stir gently until the chicken is fully coated.

4 Scoop the dressed chicken over the greens and serve with the sesame seeds sprinkled over the top.

Smoked Trout Salad

281 calories

4
of your SIRT
5 a day

Trout (and in fact all oily fish) is a great source of SIRTs.

Serves 2 • *Ready in 20 minutes*

200g new potatoes, halved
50g rocket
50g young spinach leaves
50g watercress

8 radishes, trimmed and quartered

Large handful (20g) parsley, roughly chopped

100g red seedless grapes, halved

130g smoked trout, cut into thin slices

For the dressing:

1 tbsp mayonnaise

1 tbsp natural yogurt

1 tsp olive oil

2 tsp capers, chopped

2 cocktail gherkins, finely chopped

Juice of ½ lemon

1 Steam the new potatoes for 15–20 minutes until tender.
2 In a large bowl, mix together the rocket, spinach, watercress, new potatoes, radishes and parsley.
3 Stir together the mayonnaise, yogurt, olive oil, capers, gherkins and lemon juice to make the dressing. Stir half of the dressing into the greens.
4 Arrange the salad and potato over two serving plates. Distribute the grapes and smoked trout evenly between the plates. Finally drizzle over the last of the dressing.

SOUPS AND BROTHS

Soups are such versatile and warming meals. Great for a chilly day. And what's more, all the soups listed here can be frozen so feel free to make a big batch.

● ● ●

Proper Miso Soup

Mexican Chicken Soup

Thai Spinach Soup

Savoy Cabbage and Bacon Soup

Edamame Bean and Pesto Soup

Spicy Butternut Squash and Kale Soup

Kale and Stilton Soup

Slow Onion Soup

Parsley Soup

Greens in Curried Broth

Proper Miso Soup

88 calories

3
of your SIRT
5 a day

A real miso soup is bursting with flavour – and SIRTs – and is filling yet low calorie. If you can, I strongly recommend making it a part of your SIRT diet. It is absolutely perfect for your jump-start days.

Although the soup takes only 10 minutes to make, the proper ingredients require a trip to an Asian supermarket or top-notch health-food store. The key ingredient is the miso paste and the stuff you can buy in supermarkets just isn't a patch on the real thing. None of the ingredients are expensive – you can buy a whole week's worth for under 10 pounds. I like my local Asian market but I have also used the excellent Japan Centre (www.japancentre.com) to find everything I need and more. The specialist ingredients needed are: white miso paste, wakame (dried seaweed) and dashi stock powder (Japanese fish stock). You also need tofu, which can be bought just about anywhere.

Finally, the key to a good miso soup is to never ever boil the miso paste. Bear that in mind as the most important part of the process. ☞

Serves 2–3 • Ready in 10 minutes

10g wakame
1 litre water
5g (1 sachet) instant dashi granules
100g tofu, chopped into cubes
1 heaped tbsp (25g) white miso paste
2 spring onions, trimmed and chopped

1 Place the wakame in a small bowl or cup and generously cover with water. Leave to soak for a few minutes.
2 Bring the 1 litre water to the boil in a large saucepan. Stir in the instant dashi powder until dissolved. Turn the heat down to a simmer and add the tofu. Remove the wakame from the soaking liquor and, discarding the water, add the wakame to the soup. Cook for 2 minutes.
3 Place the miso paste in a bowl and add some of the dashi broth a tablespoon at a time, stirring until the miso has dissolved and you have a smooth thick sauce.
4 Remove the saucepan from the heat and then stir in the miso. Taste the soup and add a little more miso if desired.
5 Serve in two bowls, sprinkling the chopped spring onion equally over each dish.

Mexican Chicken Soup

361 calories

2
of your SIRT
5 a day

This soup is thick and very tasty. All the beans add plenty of SIRTs to the meal.

Serves 4 • Ready in 55 minutes

4 chicken drumsticks

2 shallots, peeled and roughly chopped

1 carrot, peeled and roughly chopped

1 litre water

400g tin chopped tomatoes

300ml passata

1 green pepper, deseeded and chopped

1 red chilli, deseeded and finely chopped

2 cloves garlic, peeled and crushed

1 tsp dried mixed herbs

1 tsp paprika

1 tsp smoked paprika

½ tsp ground turmeric

½ tsp ground cumin

1 tsp mild chilli powder

400g tin black beans, drained

400g tin kidney beans, drained

30g (very large handful) flat-leaf parsley, chopped

Salt and freshly ground black pepper

1 Place the chicken drumsticks, shallots and carrot in a large saucepan. Pour over the water and bring up to a simmer. Cook for 20 minutes, then remove the chicken drumsticks with a slotted spoon and set aside to cool.

2 Add the chopped tomatoes, passata, green pepper, chilli and garlic and bring back up to simmering point. Add the dried herbs, paprika, smoked paprika, turmeric, cumin and chilli powder, then simmer gently for 30 minutes.

3 Remove the skin from the drumsticks and pull as much chicken as possible off the bone. Shred the chicken meat and return it to the pan, along with the black beans and kidney beans, for the last 5 minutes of cooking. Remove from the heat and stir in the parsley. Season generously with salt and pepper.

Thai Spinach Soup

228 calories

2
of your SIRT
5 a day

There's something very comforting about this recipe, like a warm and spicy blanket. You can add rice or chicken (or both!) to the soup to make it more of a meal.

Serves 4 • *Ready in 20 minutes*

1 tsp olive oil

2 shallots, peeled and chopped

½ tsp ground cumin

1 thumb (5cm) fresh ginger, peeled and grated

1 stick lemongrass

1 red chilli, deseeded if preferred, chopped

Zest and juice of 1 lime (washed in hot soapy
water to remove wax first)

1 litre boiling water

400g tin coconut milk

250g fresh spinach

1 tbsp Thai green curry paste

Large handful (20g) parsley, stalks discarded
and roughly chopped

Large handful (20g) coriander, stalks discarded
and roughly chopped

1 In a large saucepan, heat the olive oil gently and fry the shallots for 5 minutes until starting to soften. Add the cumin, fresh ginger, lemongrass, chilli and lime zest. Stir through, then pour in the water. Bring up to the boil, then add the coconut milk, return to a gentle simmer and cook for a further 10 minutes.

2 Add the spinach and curry paste and simmer gently until the spinach has cooked through. Remove from the heat and discard the lemongrass stick. Stir in the parsley, coriander and lime juice.

Savoy Cabbage and Bacon Soup

296 calories

2
of your SIRT
5 a day

Savoy cabbage contains lots of SIRTs, so makes a filling soup for a cold winter's day.

Serves 6 • Ready in 30 minutes

200g bacon or pancetta, roughly chopped
2 shallots, peeled and chopped
2 cloves garlic, peeled and sliced
200g white potatoes, peeled and roughly chopped
1.2 litres boiling water
500ml chicken stock, fresh or made with 1 cube
1 tsp English mustard
800g savoy cabbage (1 small or ½ large), stalk removed and shredded
200ml crème fraîche
Very large handful (30g) parsley, roughly chopped

1 Heat a large saucepan at a high temperature and toss in the bacon. Fry for 3–5 minutes, turning regularly, until browned and crispy. Remove with a slotted spoon and set aside. Add the shallots, stir and turn the heat down to low. Cook the shallots for 5 minutes.

2 Add the garlic and potato, fry for a few minutes, then add the boiling water, chicken stock and mustard. Bring back to the boil and simmer for 10 minutes. Add the cabbage, return to boiling and cook for another 6 minutes.

3 Transfer to a blender in two batches and blend until smooth. Reintroduce the bacon and reheat the soup gently in the pan. When lightly bubbling, add the crème fraîche and cook for 2 more minutes before serving.

Edamame Bean and Pesto Soup

272 calories

1½
of your SIRT
5 a day

A rich, thick and very green soup.

Serves 2 • Ready in 40 minutes

1 tsp olive oil
1 leek, trimmed and sliced
1 clove garlic, peeled and sliced
100g white potatoes, peeled and diced
200g fresh or frozen soya/edamame beans
3-4 basil leaves, torn
750ml vegetable stock, fresh or made with 1 cube
50g baby leaf spinach, torn
1 tbsp pesto

1 Heat the oil in a large saucepan and gently fry the leek and garlic for 10 minutes. Add the potato, three-quarters of the soya beans and the basil. Add the stock, bring back to the boil and simmer gently for 20 minutes.

2 Transfer the soup to a blender and blend until smooth. Return the soup to the pan and bring to a gentle simmer. Stir in the rest of the soya beans, the spinach and pesto and heat for a further 5 minutes.

Spicy Butternut Squash and Kale Soup

340 calories

2½
of your SIRT
5 a day

This vegetarian soup is thick and creamy.

Serves 4   •   Ready in 45 minutes

1 tbsp olive oil

2 shallots, peeled and chopped

1 clove garlic, peeled and sliced

200g sweet potato, peeled and diced

800g (1 small) butternut squash, deseeded, peeled and diced

1 red chilli, deseeded and chopped

1 tsp smoked paprika

½ tsp paprika

1 tsp ground turmeric

1 tsp salt

500ml vegetable stock, fresh or made with 1 cube

1 litre boiling water

1 tbsp wholegrain mustard

20g Parmesan cheese, finely grated

200g kale leaves, stalks removed and
roughly chopped

200ml crème fraîche

1 Heat the oil in a large heavy-bottomed saucepan. Toss in the shallots and garlic and stir-fry for 5 minutes. Add the sweet potato and butternut squash. Stir, cover and cook gently for 10 minutes. Stir in the chilli, both paprikas, turmeric and salt. Add the stock and water and bring to the boil. Simmer for 20 minutes.

2 Transfer to a blender in two batches and blend until smooth. Return to the pan and reheat gently. Add the mustard, Parmesan cheese and kale. Cook for 5 minutes until the kale is tender. Add the crème fraîche, bring back to temperature and serve.

Kale and Stilton Soup

266 calories

3
of your SIRT
5 a day

This soup also tastes good with savoy cabbage or for something a little bit different, try red cabbage.

Serves 4 • Ready in 45 minutes

1 tbsp olive oil
2 shallots, peeled and diced
2 leeks, trimmed and sliced
150g white potatoes, peeled and diced
500ml vegetable stock, fresh or made with 1 cube
500ml boiling water
400g kale leaves, stalks removed and roughly chopped
2 tbsp (30ml) sherry
200ml semi-skimmed milk
2 tbsp (30ml) double cream
50g Stilton, crumbled
Large handful (20g) curly parsley, roughly chopped
Salt and freshly ground black pepper

1 Heat the oil in a large saucepan and gently fry the shallots and leek for 10 minutes until tender. Stir in the potato,

then add the stock and boiling water. Bring to the boil, then reduce the heat and simmer gently for 15 minutes. Use a potato masher to mash the potatoes in the pan – or blend in a blender if you prefer.

2 Add the kale, bring to a gentle simmer and cook for 4 minutes until the kale is just tender. Add the sherry, milk, cream and half the Stilton. Simmer until the Stilton has all dissolved. Season generously with salt and pepper. Divide into four bowls and serve with parsley and Stilton sprinkled over.

Slow Onion Soup

219 calories

3
of your SIRT
5 a day

Cook the onions long and slow to allow the natural sweetness of the onions to shine through.

Serves 4 • Ready in 1½ hours

1 tbsp olive oil
20g butter
1kg white onions, peeled and finely sliced
1 clove garlic, peeled and sliced
2 leaves thyme, finely chopped (or 1 tsp dried thyme)

☞

1 bay leaf
1 tsp salt
200ml red wine
1 litre fresh beef stock
40g flat-leaf parsley, roughly chopped
1 tsp sugar
Freshly ground black pepper

1 Heat the oil and butter gently in a wide lidded frying pan. When the butter has melted, add the onion, garlic, thyme, bay leaf and salt.

2 On the smallest ring, with the heat on the lowest possible setting, put the lid on the pan (slightly askew to allow a little steam to escape) and cook for about 1 hour, stirring occasionally.

3 Add the wine, beef stock, parsley and sugar, then bring to the boil, reduce the heat and simmer for 30 minutes. Serve with a generous seasoning of black pepper.

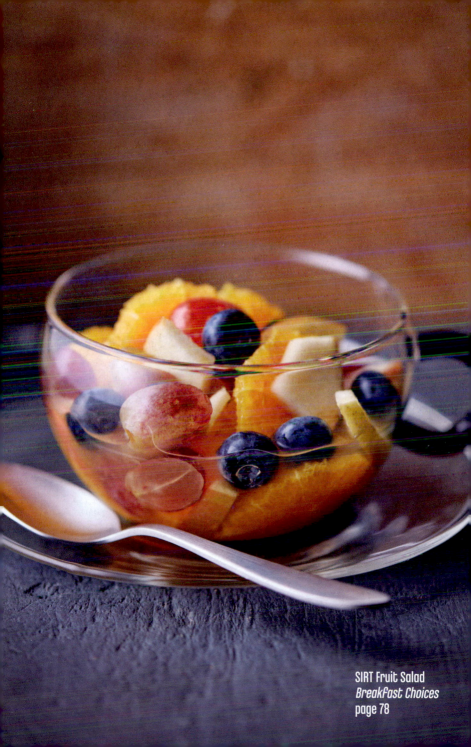

SIRT Fruit Salad
Breakfast Choices
page 78

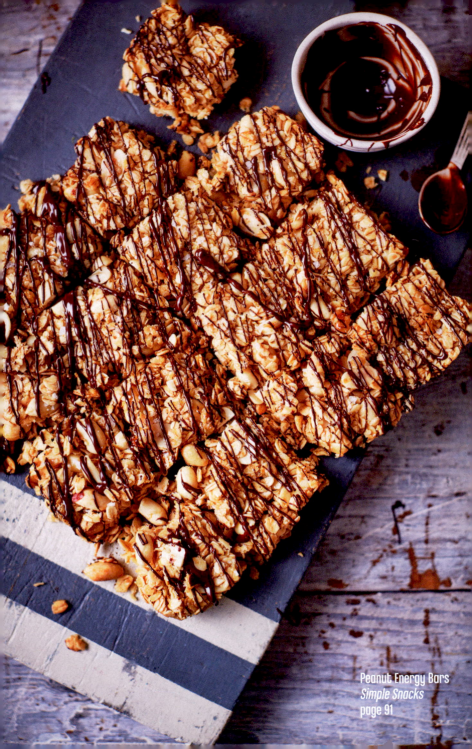

Peanut Energy Bars
Simple Snacks
page 91

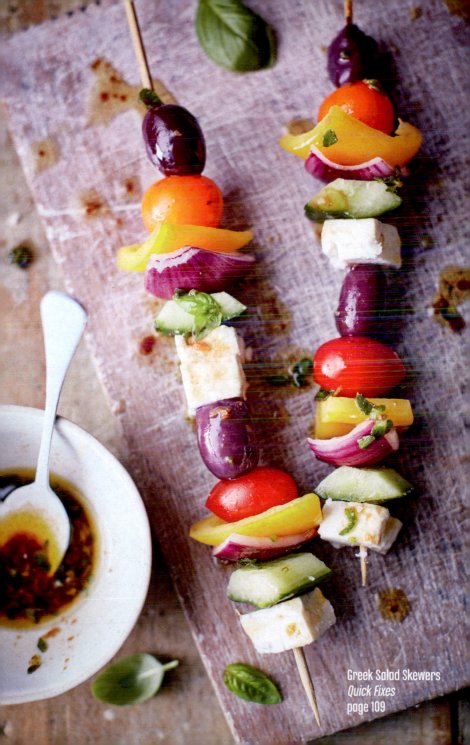

Greek Salad Skewers
Quick Fixes
page 109

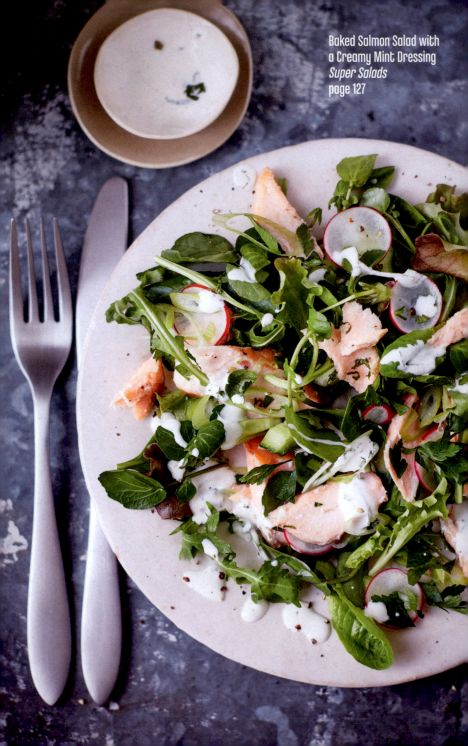

Baked Salmon Salad with
a Creamy Mint Dressing
Super Salads
page 127

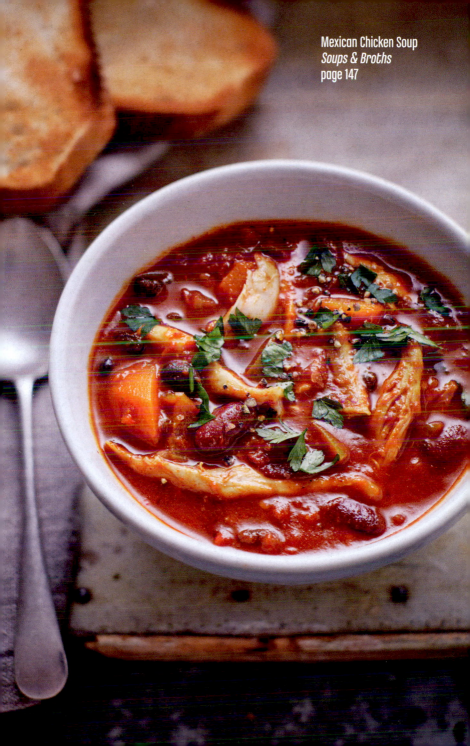

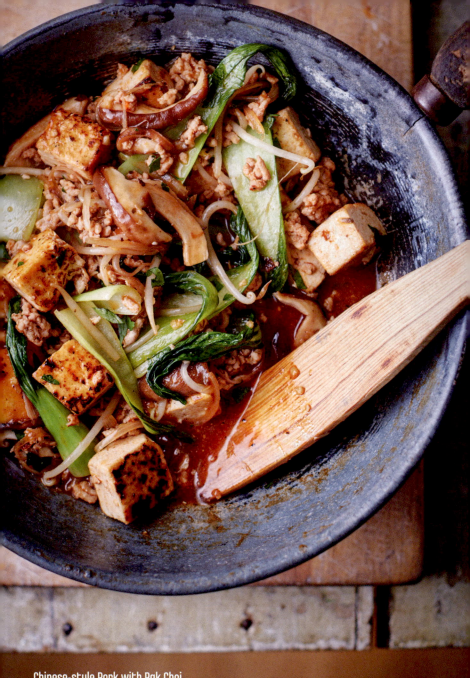

Chinese-style Pork with Pak Choi
Main Meals
page 196

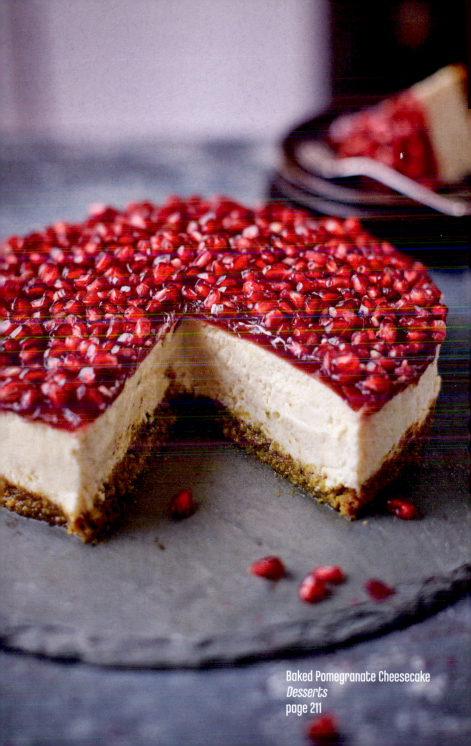

Baked Pomegranate Cheesecake
Desserts
page 211

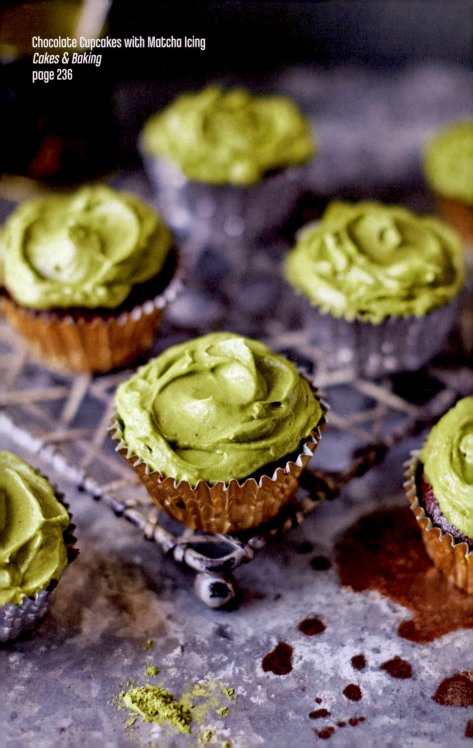

Chocolate Cupcakes with Matcha Icing
Cakes & Baking
page 236

Parsley Soup

232 calories

3
of your SIRT
5 a day

You can use flat-leaf or curly parsley in this recipe.

Serves 4 • Ready in 25 minutes

1 tbsp olive oil

4 shallots, peeled and chopped

700g white potatoes, peeled and diced

100g parsley, stalks and leaves divided, roughly chopped

400ml fresh chicken or vegetable stock

1 litre boiling water

Salt and freshly ground black pepper

4 heaped tsp (10g each) crème fraîche

1 Heat the oil on a low heat in a large heavy bottomed saucepan. Add the shallots and cook gently for 5–10 minutes until soft but not browned. Add the potatoes and the parsley stalks, stir, then add the stock and water. Bring to the boil and simmer for 15 minutes.

2 Remove from the heat and stir in the rest of the parsley. Blend, in two batches if necessary, until smooth. Return to the heat and bring back to a simmer for 2–3 minutes. Season generously with salt and pepper. Serve with a teaspoon of crème fraîche swirled into the top of each bowl.

Greens in Curried Broth

130 calories

3
of your SIRT
5 a day

This low-calorie broth packs a bit of a punch. If you prefer it less hot and spicy, reduce the chilli by half.

Serves 4 • Ready in 25 minutes

1 tbsp olive oil

2 shallots, peeled and finely chopped

1 clove garlic, peeled and finely chopped

2 green chillies, deseeded and finely chopped

1 tsp mild chilli powder

1 tsp ground turmeric

¼ tsp cloves

¼ tsp ground cinnamon

1 tsp salt

150g broccoli, cut into small florets

200g kale leaves, stalks removed and roughly chopped

400ml chicken or vegetable stock,
fresh or made with 1 cube

1 litre boiling water

250g tofu, cut into small cubes

2 spring onions, trimmed and chopped

20g coriander, chopped

1 Heat the oil on a low heat in a large heavy-bottomed saucepan. Add the shallots and stir-fry for 5 minutes until just starting to soften. Add the garlic, green chilli, spices and salt. Stir, then add the broccoli and kale. Stir-fry for 2–3 minutes. Add the stock and water and bring to the boil. Simmer gently for 15 minutes.

2 Add the tofu, spring onions and coriander and cook for a few more minutes until warmed through.

SPEEDY SUPPERS

Ready in less than 20 minutes. Perfect
for midweek meals.

• • •

Grilled Chicken with Lemon and Olives

Spiced Salmon with Potatoes and Rocket

Turmeric Prawns

Quick Vegetable Stir-Fry with Black-Bean Sauce

Beef and Broccoli

Soy-Glazed Salmon

Tandoori Spears

Fresh Saag Paneer

Fragrant Asian Hotpot

Quick-Fried Beef with Salsa Verde

Teriyaki Salmon with Chinese Vegetables

Kale and Tomato Pasta

One-Pot Curry and Rice

Grilled Chicken with Lemon and Olives

270 calories

2
of your SIRT
5 a day

This simple recipe is made by marinating the chicken in the lemon marinade after cooking. Serve with new potatoes and a green salad.

Serves 2 • Ready in 20 minutes

2 skinless chicken breast fillets
1 tsp olive oil
Zest and juice of 1 lemon (washed in hot soapy water to remove wax first)
½ clove garlic, peeled and crushed
50g good-quality large green olives, pitted and halved
1 tbsp extra virgin olive oil
1 tsp balsamic vinegar
Large handful (20g) parsley, finely chopped
Salt and freshly ground black pepper

1 Turn on the grill to a medium-high setting.
2 Cut the chicken breasts in half widthways. Make another cut into the thickest part of each chicken piece. The cut should be about an inch long and go about halfway through

the meat. This makes the chicken piece bigger and flatter and allows it to cook more evenly. Rub each piece with a little olive oil and place them all on the grill tray. Cook for between 10 and 20 minutes, turning halfway through cooking, so that the chicken is browned on the outside and cooked through. The size of the chicken pieces and the huge variation from grill to grill makes it hard to set an exact time. Obviously this dish also works well with other methods of cooking including the barbecue.

3 Meanwhile prepare the marinade in a shallow dish that can hold the chicken pieces lying flat. Simply place the lemon zest and juice, garlic, halved olives, extra virgin olive oil, balsamic vinegar, chopped parsley and a generous seasoning of salt and pepper straight into the serving dish. Roughly stir together.

4 When the chicken is cooked, transfer immediately to the serving dish and turn each piece so that it is fully covered in the sauce. Leave to rest in the dish for 2–3 minutes before serving, drizzling any remaining marinade over the chicken as you serve.

Spiced Salmon with Potatoes and Rocket

407 calories

3
of your SIRT
5 a day

This dish is very easy to make and the flavours combine beautifully. You can use tinned or fresh salmon here so it's a great store cupboard standby.

Serves 1 • Ready in 25 minutes

4 new potatoes, quartered
1 tsp olive oil
125g cooked salmon, lightly flaked
½ tsp ground turmeric
½ tsp mild chilli powder
¼ tsp ground cinnamon
Salt and freshly ground black pepper
1 tsp capers
40g rocket leaves
Handful (10g) parsley, roughly chopped
Juice of ½ lemon

1 Steam the new potatoes for 15–20 minutes until tender. Drain.

2 Heat the oil in a frying pan on a medium heat. Add the new potatoes and fry for 3–4 minutes, stirring once,

until browned. Add the salmon, turmeric, chilli powder, cinnamon and salt and pepper and fry for 2 more minutes until cooked through. Remove from the heat and stir through the capers, rocket leaves, parsley and lemon juice. Serve immediately.

Turmeric Prawns

414 calories

3
of your SIRT
5 a day

This is a vibrant and tasty dish.

Serves 2   •   Ready in 20 minutes

1 tsp olive oil
½ tsp cumin seeds
½ cinnamon stick
2 cloves
1 bay leaf
1 small red onion, chopped
1 red pepper, deseeded and chopped
2 cloves garlic, peeled and thinly sliced
1 red or green chilli, deseeded and sliced
½ tsp mild chilli powder
1 tsp paprika

1 tsp ground turmeric
½ tsp salt
2 fresh tomatoes, roughly chopped
60g frozen soya/edamame beans
1 tbsp water
250g cooked king prawns (if frozen, defrost as per the packet instructions before use)
250g cooked and cooled basmati rice
50g rocket

1 In a wide lidded frying pan, heat the oil on a medium heat. Add the cumin seeds, cinnamon stick, cloves and bay leaf. Fry for 1 minute before adding the onion and red pepper. Stir, turn the heat to low and place the lid on the pan. Cook for 5 minutes.

2 Remove the lid from the pan. Add the garlic, chilli, chilli powder, paprika, turmeric and salt and fry for a further minute. Add the chopped tomatoes, soya beans and water. Replace the lid on the pan and cook gently for 7 minutes.

3 Take the lid off the pan and remove the cinnamon stick, cloves and bay leaf. Add the prawns and rice and cook for 3–4 minutes until warmed. Finally, stir through the rocket just before serving.

Quick Vegetable Stir-Fry with Black-Bean Sauce

343 calories

4
of your SIRT
5 a day

A tasty, easy vegetarian dinner.

Serves 2   •   Ready in 10 minutes

250g firm tofu, cut into large cubes
100g cooked black beans, rinsed and drained
2 heaped tsp (30g) blackcurrant jam
½ tsp ground ginger
1 tbsp dark soy sauce
1 tsp cornflour
salt and freshly ground black pepper
1 tbsp rapeseed oil
1 shallot, peeled and cut into thin slices
¼ savoy cabbage, stalk removed and cut into thin slices
100g curly kale, stalks removed and cut thinly
1 large carrot, peeled and cut into matchsticks
100g beansprouts

1 Spread the tofu out on a plate covered in kitchen paper. Cover with kitchen paper and set aside.
2 Place the black beans, blackcurrant jam, ginger, soy sauce and cornflour into a food processor and blend until smooth.

3 Season the tofu generously with the salt and pepper. Heat the oil in a wide frying pan or wok. On a high heat, stir-fry the tofu until golden brown all over. Remove from the pan with a slotted spoon and set aside. Add the shallot, cabbage, kale and carrot to the pan and stir-fry for 3–4 minutes. Add the beansprouts and fry for 2 more minutes.

4 Reduce the heat to medium-low and return the tofu to the pan. Add the black-bean sauce and warm through for 2 minutes before serving.

Beef and Broccoli

409 calories

2
of your SIRT
5 a day

A fab quick-and-easy supper.

Serves 2 • Ready in 15 minutes

1 tbsp cornflour
1 tbsp water
1 clove garlic, peeled and crushed
250g frying steak, cut into thin strips
2 tsp rapeseed oil
1 small red onion, cut into wedges
1 small head broccoli, cut into small florets
2 tbsp soy sauce

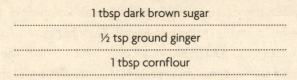

| 1 tbsp dark brown sugar |
| ½ tsp ground ginger |
| 1 tbsp cornflour |

1 Mix together the cornflour, water and garlic and stir until smooth. Add the steak and stir until thoroughly coated. Heat the oil in a shallow wide frying pan on a high heat. When hot, toss in the beef and quick fry until it's just cooked (or however you like your steak cooked). Remove from the pan with a slotted spoon and set aside.

2 Add the onion and broccoli to the pan, toss through, reduce the heat a little and cook for 4–5 minutes until tender with a little bit of bite in the broccoli.

3 Mix the soy sauce, brown sugar, ginger and cornflour together until smooth. Return the beef to the pan and add the soy sauce mixture. Stir well and cook through for a further 2 minutes.

Soy-Glazed Salmon

322 calories

1½
of your SIRT
5 a day

This is one of my favourite everyday suppers. It's so quick and easy to cook. Serve on a bed of freshly cooked kale.

Serves 2 • Ready in 15 minutes

2 tbsp soy sauce

1 tbsp balsamic vinegar

½ tsp chilli flakes

1 small thumb (3cm) fresh ginger, peeled and finely grated

1 tbsp honey

½ clove garlic, peeled and crushed

2 × 150g salmon fillets, skin on

1 tsp olive oil

1 Place the soy, balsamic, chilli flakes, ginger, honey and garlic in a wide bowl and whisk together with a fork until the honey has dissolved. Place the salmon fillets in the bowl skin side up and leave to rest for 2–3 minutes.

2 Heat the oil in a frying pan on a medium-high heat. When hot, put the salmon in, but not the marinade, cooking them skin side up. Cook for 5–6 minutes. Use a fish slice to turn the salmon over so it is skin side down. Turn the heat down to low. After a minute (or when the heat has reduced) pour the remaining marinade around the fish. When gently bubbling cook for a further 5 minutes or until the fish is cooked through. Serve with the sauce dribbled over the fish.

Tandoori Spears

240 calories

4
of your SIRT
5 a day

This can be cooked under the grill or it makes a great vegetarian barbecue dish.

Serves 2 • Ready in 15 minutes

4 wooden skewers, soaked in water for 30 minutes before use
400g firm tofu, cut into large cubes
3 tsp tandoori masala powder (dry tandoori spice mix)
1 tsp ground turmeric
Juice of 1 lime
salt and freshly ground black pepper
1 red onion, cut into large slices
1 red pepper, deseeded and cut into large pieces
100g natural yogurt
Large bunch (20g) parsley, roughly chopped

1 Spread the tofu out on a plate covered in kitchen paper. Cover with kitchen paper and set aside.

2 Mix the tandoori masala, turmeric, lime juice and plenty of salt and pepper together. Add the tofu pieces, stir until fully coated and leave to rest for 5 minutes.

3 Heat the grill/barbecue to high. Cover the grill tray with a piece of foil (turned up at the edges to catch juices).

4 Prepare four equal skewers by threading on a piece of onion, tofu and red pepper. You should get two sets of onion, tofu and red pepper on each skewer. Make sure the ingredients are not too squashed together.

5 Mix the remaining marinade with the yogurt and fresh parsley. Gently brush this onto all of the skewers on all sides. Place on the prepared grill tray. Place under the hot grill for approximately 5 minutes until browned on one side, then turn and cook for another 5 minutes until cooked through and the vegetables are softened and slightly charred.

Fresh Saag Paneer

279 calories

3
of your SIRT
5 a day

Using fresh spinach gives a whole new dimension (and lots of SIRTs) to this curry-house favourite.

Serves 2 • Ready in 20 minutes

2 tsp rapeseed oil
200g paneer, cut into cubes
Salt and freshly ground black pepper
1 red onion, chopped
1 small thumb (3cm) fresh ginger, peeled and cut into matchsticks

1 clove garlic, peeled and thinly sliced

1 green chilli, deseeded and finely sliced

100g cherry tomatoes, halved

½ tsp ground coriander

½ tsp ground cumin

¼ tsp ground turmeric

½ tsp mild chilli powder

½ tsp salt

100g fresh spinach leaves

Small handful (10g) parsley, chopped

Small handful (10g) coriander, chopped

1 Heat the oil in a wide lidded frying pan over a high heat. Season the paneer generously with salt and pepper and toss into the pan. Fry for a few minutes until golden, stirring often. Remove from the pan with a slotted spoon and set aside.

2 Reduce the heat and add the onion. Fry for 5 minutes before adding the ginger, garlic and chilli. Cook for another couple of minutes before adding the cherry tomatoes. Put the lid on the pan and cook for a further 5 minutes.

3 Add the spices and salt, then stir. Return the paneer to the pan and stir until coated. Add the spinach to the pan together with the parsley and coriander and put the lid on. Allow the spinach to wilt for 1–2 minutes, then incorporate into the dish. Serve immediately.

Fragrant Asian Hotpot

185 calories

1½
of your SIRT
5 a day

This is a light and tasty Asian dish.

Serves 2 • *Ready in 15 minutes*

1 tsp tomato purée

1 star anise, crushed (or ¼ tsp ground anise)

Small handful (10g) parsley, stalks finely chopped

Small handful (10g) coriander, stalks finely chopped

Juice of ½ lime

500ml chicken stock, fresh or made with 1 cube

½ carrot, peeled and cut into matchsticks

50g broccoli, cut into small florets

50g beansprouts

100g raw tiger prawns

100g firm tofu, chopped

50g rice noodles, cooked according to
packet instructions

50g cooked water chestnuts, drained

20g sushi ginger, chopped

1 tbsp good-quality miso paste

1 Place the tomato purée, star anise, parsley stalks, coriander stalks, lime juice and chicken stock in a large pan and bring to a simmer for 10 minutes.

2 Add the carrot, broccoli, prawns, tofu, noodles and water chestnuts and simmer gently until the prawns are cooked through. Remove from the heat and stir in the sushi ginger and miso paste.

3 Serve sprinkled with the parsley and coriander leaves.

Quick-Fried Beef with Salsa Verde

335 calories

2
of your SIRT
5 a day

The salsa verde tastes even better if prepared in advance and left to rest in the fridge for an hour or so before cooking.

Serves 2 • Ready in 15 minutes

10g flat-leaf parsley, finely chopped
2 leaves basil, chopped
2 leaves mint, chopped
2 cocktail gherkins, finely chopped
1 tsp capers, drained
2 anchovy fillets, drained and chopped
1 tsp red wine vinegar

Juice of ½ lime
1 tsp Dijon mustard
1 tsp extra virgin olive oil
100g broccoli, cut into small florets
2 × 150g beef escalopes
Salt and freshly ground black pepper
1 tsp rapeseed oil
1 clove garlic, peeled and thinly sliced

1 Place the parsley, basil, mint, gherkins, capers, anchovies, vinegar, lime juice, Dijon mustard and extra virgin olive oil in a bowl and stir together. Cover and leave to rest for at least 5 minutes.

2 Steam the broccoli over a pan of boiling water for 5 minutes or until just tender.

3 Wrap the beef lightly in clingfilm and beat with a rolling pin until about half a centimetre thick. Remove from the clingfilm and season on both sides with the salt and pepper.

4 Heat the rapeseed oil in a wide lidded frying pan to a high heat. Add the garlic, stir, then immediately add the beef. Fry for just 1–2 minutes on each side. Turn off the heat, stir in the broccoli, place the lid on the pan and leave to rest for 3–5 minutes. Serve with the salsa verde drizzled over.

Teriyaki Salmon with Chinese Vegetables

354 calories

2½
of your SIRT
5 a day

The salmon in this dish is steamed rather than baked, which gives it a more delicate taste and texture.

Serves 2 • Ready in 15 minutes

1 thumb (5cm) fresh ginger, peeled and grated
1 tbsp soy sauce
1 tsp fish sauce
1 tsp honey
1 tsp sesame oil
2 salmon fillets, skinless, quartered
1 shallot, peeled and thinly sliced
½ carrot, peeled and cut into sticks
1 bulb fennel, thinly sliced
1 bulb pak choi, sliced
100g kale leaves, stalks removed and torn

1 Stir the ginger, soy, fish sauce, honey and sesame oil together in a wide bowl. Place the salmon pieces in the bowl, turning and covering each piece in the sauce. Leave to rest while you prepare the rest of the meal.

2 In a large lidded frying pan add about 5mm–1 cm depth of water and bring to the boil. Add the shallot, carrot and fennel. Place the lid on the pan and cook for 4 minutes. Add the pak choi and kale, stir through lightly and add a little more water if the pan looks dry. Arrange the pieces of salmon on top of vegetables and pour in any remaining marinade. Return the lid to the pan and steam for 8 minutes until the salmon is cooked through.

Kale and Tomato Pasta

520 calories

5
of your SIRT
5 a day

This ridiculously easy dish can be made in less than 10 minutes.

Serves 2 • Ready in 10 minutes

200g linguine
200g cherry tomatoes, halved
Zest of 1 lemon (washed in hot soapy water to remove wax first)
Juice of ½ lemon
50ml extra virgin olive oil
1 heaped tsp sea salt
500ml boiling water

☞

200g kale leaves, stalks removed and roughly torn
Large handful (20g) parsley, finely chopped
20g Parmesan, finely grated
Freshly ground black pepper

1 Use a large lidded shallow pan, wide enough to hold the linguine lying flat. Place the pasta, tomatoes, lemon zest, lemon juice, olive oil and salt in the pan. Pour over 500ml boiling water, put the lid on and bring to the boil.

2 As soon as it is boiling, remove the lid and stir. Continue to boil, stirring every minute, for 6 minutes. Add the kale and cook for a further 2 minutes or until almost all of the water has evaporated.

3 Combine the parsley, Parmesan and black pepper in a small bowl.

4 Divide the pasta between two bowls and sprinkle the parsley and Parmesan mixture over.

One-Pot Curry and Rice

347 calories

2
of your SIRT
5 a day

Try using pouches of cooked rice and lentils to make this dish really quick and easy. This dish is equally good served as a cold lunch the next day.

Serves 4 • Ready in 20 minutes

2 tsp rapeseed oil

225g paneer, cut into cubes

Salt and freshly ground black pepper

1 red onion, sliced

1 thumb (5cm) fresh ginger, peeled and grated

2 cloves garlic, peeled and grated

2 finger chillies, heads removed and finely
chopped with the seeds in

½ tsp aniseed seeds

250g cooked brown rice

250g ready-to-eat or cooked puy lentils

100g frozen soya/edamame beans

½ tsp salt

½ tsp ground turmeric

½ tsp ground cumin

½ tsp ground coriander

1 tsp mild chilli powder

2 tomatoes, roughly chopped

50g baby leaf spinach

Large handful (20g) parsley, chopped

1 Heat the oil in a large frying pan on a high heat and add
   the paneer. Season generously with salt and pepper. Cook
   the paneer, stirring frequently, until golden brown all
   over. Remove with a slotted spoon and set aside.

2 Add the onion and then reduce the heat in the pan to
   low. Cook for 2 minutes before adding the ginger, garlic,
   chillies and aniseed and leave to cook slowly for a further
   5 minutes. ☞

3 Tip the rice and lentils into a large bowl and mix together gently, breaking up clumps and separating grains as you do so.

4 If the soya beans are frozen or require cooking, cook as per the packet instructions.

5 Add the salt, ground spices and chilli powder to the frying pan and stir. Add the rice and lentil mixture, soya beans and tomatoes to the pan. Stir very well and cook through until piping hot. Finally add the spinach, parsley and return the paneer to the pan. Stir to combine, then serve immediately.

6 Any spare portions, once fully cooled, can be refrigerated and served cold the next day.

MAIN MEALS

For when you are after a proper sit-down meal,
with or without your family.

• • •

Tandoori Chicken and Peas

Mini Turkey Burgers with Parsley Salad

Creamy Fish Pie

Spinach and Feta Quiche with Buckwheat Crust

Cauliflower Curry

Chicken and Lemon Tagine with Herby Rice

Chinese-Style Pork with Pak Choi

Chicken with Pesto Crust

Chicken and Watercress Pie

Kale, Edamame and Tofu Curry

Beef in Red Wine with Kale Mashed Potato

Cheesy Greens Pasta Bake

Sticky Pork with Apple

Tandoori Chicken and Peas

461 calories

4
of your SIRT
5 a day

This totally flavoursome dish is warming, healthy and very filling.

Serves 2 • Ready in 40 minutes + 1–2 hours marinating time

Juice of 1 lemon

2 tsp tandoori masala powder (dry tandoori spice mix)

1 tsp ground turmeric

2 × 150g skinless chicken breast fillets,
cut into large pieces

300g new potatoes

150g fresh or frozen soya/edamame beans

2 tsp olive oil

2 shallots, peeled and finely diced

1 red chilli, deseeded and cut into rings

1 green pepper, deseeded and chopped

2 cloves garlic, peeled and thinly sliced

30g parsley, roughly chopped

Salt and freshly ground black pepper

1 Place the lemon juice and spices in a wide bowl. Add the chicken and turn through the marinade until fully coated. Cover and refrigerate for at least an hour.

2 Steam the new potatoes for 18–20 minutes until tender. If the soya beans are frozen or require cooking, cook as per the packet instructions.

3 In a large frying pan, heat the olive oil gently and add the shallots, chilli and pepper. Fry slowly for 5 minutes. Turn the heat up to medium and add the chicken from the marinade. Do not add the marinade from the bowl, but reserve it for later. Cook the chicken for 10–14 minutes, stirring regularly until it is cooked through.

4 Add the garlic and remaining marinade and allow the sauce to bubble for a minute, then turn the heat down to low. Stir through the potatoes and soya beans and heat until warm. Remove from the heat and add the parsley. Season generously and then serve.

Mini Turkey Burgers with Parsley Salad

363 calories

3
of your SIRT
5 a day

Delicious and easy. A quick anytime favourite with myself and the kids. Normally I find turkey bland, but these burgers are delicious. The parsley salad could also be made with cooked bulgur wheat or quinoa.

Serves 4 • Ready in 30 minutes

500g turkey mince
....
Salt and freshly ground black pepper
....
1 tsp onion powder
....
1 tsp mixed dried herbs
....
1 tsp paprika
....
½ tsp ground turmeric
....
1 clove garlic, peeled and crushed
....
Handful (20g) parsley, finely chopped
....
2 tsp cornflour
....
1 tbsp olive oil

For the parsley salad:

150g couscous
....
Juice of 2 lemons
....
1 tbsp extra virgin olive oil
....
Salt and freshly ground black pepper
....
¼ tsp ground cinnamon
....
¼ tsp ground coriander
....
Pinch of ground cloves
....
Pinch of ground ginger
....
4 tomatoes, finely chopped
....
2 spring onions, finely sliced
....
100g flat-leaf parsley, stalks discarded,
leaves very finely chopped

1 To make the parsley salad, place the couscous in a bowl and add the lemon juice, extra virgin olive oil and plenty of salt and pepper. Add all the spices, erring on the side of caution, especially with the cinnamon and cloves. Stir to combine. Pour over enough water to generously cover the couscous. Leave to rest for approximately 10 minutes until all the water is absorbed and the couscous has swelled and is cooked 'al dente'. Top up the water a little at a time as needed during the rest period.

2 Meanwhile combine the tomato, spring onion and parsley. Mix the salad into the spicy couscous and allow to meld for at least 5 minutes before serving.

3 Place the turkey mince in a large bowl and add a generous seasoning of salt and pepper, the onion powder, dried herbs, paprika, turmeric, garlic, parsley and cornflour. Mix together well with your hands, breaking up the strands of mince as you go.

4 When thoroughly mixed, pull out ping-pong ball-sized lumps of the mix, roll gently into balls, then flatten slightly by pressing gently into the palm of your hand. Place the burgers on a plate. The mixture should make 12 to 14 small burgers.

5 Heat the oil in a large wide pan and when hot spread the burgers out in the pan. Leave to cook undisturbed for 4 minutes, turn with a slotted spoon and cook for a further 4 minutes. Serve the burgers with the parsley salad.

Creamy Fish Pie

359 calories

2
of your SIRT
5 a day

This easy fish pie is loaded with SIRT-rich oily fish.

Serves 4 • *Ready in 30 minutes*

1 tsp olive oil

1 shallot, peeled and finely chopped

1 celery stick, trimmed and finely chopped

1 clove garlic, peeled and thinly sliced

1 × 125g salmon fillet, skinless, cut into pieces

2 × 200g pollock fillets, skinless, cut into pieces

2 × 125g small smoked trout fillets, flaked

100ml milk

1 tbsp Dijon mustard

Few sprigs dill, finely chopped

150g fresh soya/edamame beans

150ml crème fraîche

Juice of ½ lemon

Salt and freshly ground black pepper

2 slices wholemeal bread

Small handful (10g) parsley

Few leaves basil

1 Preheat the oven to 220°C (200°C fan/Gas 7).

2 In a lidded saucepan, heat the oil gently, add the shallot, celery and garlic, stir, put the lid on the pan and sweat for 5 minutes.

3 Add all the fish, milk, Dijon mustard and dill, and bring to a gentle simmer. Cook for 10 minutes, add the soya beans and cook for a further 5 minutes. Remove from the heat and stir in the crème fraîche, lemon juice and salt and pepper. Transfer to a shallow oven dish.

4 Place the bread, parsley and basil in a food processor and blitz until you have fine breadcrumbs. Sprinkle over the fish. Bake in the oven for 5 minutes or until the top is golden.

Spinach and Feta Quiche with Buckwheat Crust

494 calories

1
of your SIRT
5 a day

Using buckwheat as a crust is a great way to make a pie or a quiche without any fuss. You could also make this as a kale or watercress quiche.

Serves 4 • Ready in 1 hour

3 large eggs, at room temperature
100ml double cream
100ml crème fraîche

Pinch of grated nutmeg
½ tsp dried thyme
Freshly ground black pepper
15g butter
150g buckwheat
1 tsp olive oil
150g fresh spinach, roughly chopped
½ clove garlic, peeled and crushed
100g feta cheese, cut into small cubes

1 Preheat the oven to 190°C (170°C fan/Gas 5).

2 Place the eggs, double cream, crème fraîche, nutmeg, thyme and black pepper in a bowl and set aside.

3 Take a shallow pie dish approximately 24cm in diameter. Use the butter to thoroughly grease the dish, getting into all the corners and making sure there is a generous coating on the base and sides. Tip the buckwheat into the pie dish. Gently tip the dish and allow the buckwheat to cover and stick to the butter on the base and up the sides of the dish. Then shake a little to allow the remaining buckwheat to sit evenly on the base of the dish.

4 In a lidded pan, heat the oil gently and add the spinach and garlic. Lightly toss in the oil until sizzling. Put the lid on the pan, turn the heat off and leave to wilt for 2 minutes. Arrange the spinach over the base of the pie dish. Distribute the feta over the spinach. Now use a whisk to beat the eggs and cream together until really smooth. Pour over the spinach in the dish. ☞

5 Bake for 45 minutes or until the centre is firm with a little bit of wobble. This quiche tastes delicious hot or cold.

Cauliflower Curry

92 calories

4
of your SIRT
5 a day

This unusual vegetarian dish is full of SIRTs – cauliflower contains SIRTs too – and is filling and low calorie.

Serves 2 • Ready in 30 minutes

½ tsp ground cumin
½ tsp ground coriander
½ tsp ground turmeric
1 tsp salt
Juice of ½ lemon
2 tbsp water
1 tbsp olive oil
1 thumb (5cm) fresh ginger, peeled and cut into matchsticks
1 tsp cumin seeds
½ tsp mustard seeds
1 red onion, sliced
1 medium-sized (about 800g) cauliflower, cut into small florets
2 tomatoes, diced

1 Firstly, mix all the ground spices and salt together in a small bowl. Add the lemon juice and water.

2 In a large lidded frying pan, heat the oil on a medium heat. Quickly stir in the ginger and fry for a minute before throwing in the cumin and mustard seeds. Cook for a minute and just as they start to sizzle and pop, add in the onion and cauliflower florets. Fry for about 3–4 minutes – you want to get brown spots appearing on the cauliflower.

3 Pour the suspension of spices over the cauliflower, stir well, then turn the heat right down and put on the lid. Leave to steam for 8 minutes. Put in the diced tomatoes, stir and cook for another 10–15 minutes until the cauliflower is tender.

Chicken and Lemon Tagine with Herby Rice

489 calories

3½
of your SIRT
5 a day

A great family meal that is also suitable for guests.

Serves 4 • Ready in 2 hours

20g butter

4 chicken thighs, skin removed

1 red onion, chopped

2 cloves garlic, peeled and grated

1 thumb (5cm) fresh ginger, peeled and finely grated

1 cinnamon stick

2 tsp ras-el-hanout (North African spice blend)

1 tsp ground turmeric

1 tsp ground cinnamon

½ tsp saffron

1 preserved lemon, roughly chopped

2 tbsp honey

500ml chicken stock, fresh or made with 1 cube

100g dates, stones removed and halved

Salt and freshly ground black pepper

Large handful (30g) flat-leaf parsley,
roughly chopped

For the herby rice:

1 red onion, finely chopped

2 tomatoes, finely chopped

2 large bunches flat-leaf parsley, roughly chopped

1 bunch mint, roughly chopped

1 bunch coriander, roughly chopped

Juice of ½ lemon

Salt and freshly ground black pepper

160g brown basmati rice

1 tbsp extra virgin olive oil

1 Heat a large lidded saucepan or casserole dish on a medium heat. Add the butter and fry the chicken pieces for 2–3 minutes each side until golden brown. Remove from the pan with a slotted spoon and set aside. Add the onion, fry for 3 minutes, then add the garlic, ginger and spices and cook for 1 minute before returning the chicken to the pan and stirring until fully coated. Add the lemon, honey and stock and bring to a simmering point. Cover with the lid slightly off and cook for 1 hour.

2 Add the dates and season well with salt and pepper before cooking for another half an hour. The chicken should be tender and the sauce thickened. Remove from the heat and stir in the parsley just before serving.

3 Meanwhile, to make the herby rice, mix the red onion, tomato, herbs and lemon juice in a large bowl. Season well with salt and pepper. Leave to rest for approximately 30 minutes. Meanwhile, cook the rice (or use precooked rice) and leave to cool completely at room temperature (warning: do not leave the rice at room temperature once cooled – it is best to store it in the fridge). Separate the rice grains with a fork and add to the onion and herb mixture. Finally, stir through the olive oil. Serve the herby rice with the chicken and lemon tagine.

Chinese-Style Pork with Pak Choi

377 calories

2
of your SIRT
5 a day

Serves 4 • Ready in 25 minutes

400g firm tofu, cut into large cubes

1 tbsp cornflour

1 tbsp water

125ml chicken stock

1 tbsp rice wine

1 tbsp tomato purée

1 tsp brown sugar

1 tbsp soy sauce

1 clove garlic, peeled and crushed

1 thumb (5cm) fresh ginger, peeled and grated

1 tbsp rapeseed oil

100g shiitake mushrooms, sliced

1 shallot, peeled and sliced

200g pak choi or choi sum, cut into thin slices

400g pork mince (10% fat)

100g beansprouts

Large handful (20g) parsley, chopped

1 Lay out the tofu on kitchen paper, cover with more kitchen paper and set aside.

2 In a small bowl, mix together the cornflour and water, removing all lumps. Add the chicken stock, rice wine, tomato purée, brown sugar and soy sauce. Add the crushed garlic and ginger and stir together.

3 In a wok or large frying pan, heat the oil to a high temperature. Add the shiitake mushrooms and stir-fry for 2–3 minutes until cooked and glossy. Remove the mushrooms from the pan with a slotted spoon and set aside. Add the tofu to the pan and stir-fry until golden on all sides. Remove with a slotted spoon and set aside.

4 Add the shallot and pak choi to the wok, stir-fry for 2 minutes, then add the mince. Cook until the mince is cooked through, then add the sauce, reduce the heat a notch and allow the sauce to bubble round the meat for a minute or two. Add the beansprouts, shiitake mushrooms and tofu to the pan and warm through. Remove from the heat, stir through the parsley and serve immediately.

Chicken with Pesto Crust

311 calories

1½
of your SIRT
5 a day

A great way to jazz up some chicken.

Serves 2 • Ready in 25 minutes

20g basil
30g flat-leaf parsley
Pinch of coarse sea salt
20g pine nuts
1 tbsp extra virgin olive oil
10g Parmesan cheese, finely grated
Freshly ground black pepper
2 × 150g chicken breast fillets, skinless

1 Preheat the oven to 200°C (180°C fan/Gas 6).

2 Place the basil and parsley in a food processor with the sea salt and whizz until you have a mushy paste. Add the pine nuts and blend again, leaving the pine nuts coarse.

3 Transfer to a bowl and add the olive oil, Parmesan and black pepper. Stir together.

4 Cut the chicken fillets in half and place the four pieces on a chopping board. Cover with clingfilm and use a rolling pin to bash the chicken pieces until they are flattened to less than 1cm thick all over.

5 Place the chicken pieces on a baking tray and divide the pesto among them. Spread the pesto so that it covers the top of all the pieces evenly. Bake in the oven for approximately 20 minutes, until cooked through.

6 Serve with new potatoes and a spinach salad.

Chicken and Watercress Pie

537 calories

2
of your SIRT
5 a day

This is a hearty pie with a simple and easy breadcrumb topping.

Serves 4 • Ready in 40 minutes

250ml water
250ml milk
1 heaped tbsp plain flour
½ chicken stock cube
25g butter
Pinch of mace
Pinch of ground turmeric
1 tsp olive oil
1 red onion, diced
500g skinless and boneless chicken thighs, cut into chunks

☞

salt and freshly ground black pepper
80g watercress
150g fresh or frozen soya/edamame beans
100g panko or breadcrumbs
25g mature Cheddar cheese, grated

1 Start by placing the water, milk, flour, stock cube and butter in a saucepan and bring to the boil. Use a balloon whisk to continuously whisk the sauce from cold until thickened. When thick, remove from the heat and stir in the mace and turmeric.

2 Preheat the oven to 200°C (180°C fan/Gas 6).

3 In an ovenproof/hob-proof casserole dish, heat the oil and fry the chicken and red onion for 5 minutes. Pour in the sauce, stir and bring to a gentle simmer for 5 minutes. Taste and season with salt and pepper. Add the watercress and soya beans. Sprinkle over the panko and grated cheese. Bake for 20 minutes, or until the topping is golden brown.

Kale, Edamame and Tofu Curry

342 calories

2½
of your SIRT
5 a day

A warming and wintry curry. Easy to keep either refrigerated or frozen for another day.

Serves 4 • Ready in 45 minutes

1 tbsp rapeseed oil
1 large onion, chopped
4 cloves garlic, peeled and grated
1 large thumb (7cm) fresh ginger, peeled and grated
1 red chilli, deseeded and thinly sliced
½ tsp ground turmeric
¼ tsp cayenne pepper
1 tsp paprika
½ tsp ground cumin
1 tsp salt
250g dried red lentils
1 litre boiling water
50g frozen soya/edamame beans
200g firm tofu, chopped into cubes
2 tomatoes, roughly chopped
Juice of 1 lime
200g kale leaves, stalks removed and torn

☞

1. Put the oil in a heavy-bottomed pan over a low-medium heat. Add the onion and cook for 5 minutes before adding the garlic, ginger and chilli and cooking for a further 2 minutes. Add the turmeric, cayenne, paprika, cumin and salt. Stir through before adding the red lentils and stirring again.

2. Pour in the boiling water and bring to a hearty simmer for 10 minutes, then reduce the heat and cook for a further 20–30 minutes until the curry has a thick 'porridge' consistency.

3. Add the soya beans, tofu and tomatoes and cook for a further 5 minutes. Add the lime juice and kale leaves and cook until the kale is just tender.

Beef in Red Wine with Kale Mashed Potato

651 calories

4
of your SIRT
5 a day

A warming and healthy autumn dish.

Serves 2 • Ready in 1 hour 15 minutes

For the beef:

4 dried porcini mushrooms

2 tsp olive oil

1 shallot, peeled and finely diced

1 clove garlic, peeled and finely sliced

100g chestnut mushrooms, sliced

2 × 150g beef escalopes

200ml red wine

1 tsp cornflour

For the mash:

300g white potatoes, peeled and quartered

Salt and freshly ground black pepper

1 tsp olive oil

1 shallot, peeled and finely diced

200g kale leaves, stalks removed and torn

1 tsp Dijon mustard

1 tbsp extra virgin olive oil

1 Place the porcini mushrooms in a quarter of a cup of boiling water and leave to soak for 15 minutes.

2 Meanwhile to make the mash, place the potatoes in a large saucepan with cold water and a good pinch of salt. Turn the heat to high and cook for 30 minutes.

3 In a lidded saucepan, heat the olive oil and gently fry the shallot for 5 minutes. Add the kale, stir and place the lid on the pan. Cook for 3–4 minutes until the kale is tender. Remove from the heat and stir in the mustard.

4 When the potatoes are cooked, drain and mash with salt and pepper and the extra virgin olive oil. Add the kale and stir through. Keep it warm while you cook the beef. ☛

5 In a frying pan, heat the oil gently and add the shallot. Cook gently for 5 minutes. Turn the heat up to medium and add the garlic and mushrooms. Fry for 5 minutes, stirring occasionally, until the mushrooms are cooked and glossy. Use a slotted spoon to remove the mushroom mixture from the pan and set aside.

6 Place the beef between two pieces of clingfilm and bash with a rolling pin until it's about half as thick as the original. Turn up the heat under the pan to high and sear the beef for about 1 minute each side, then remove the beef to rest. Place the mushroom mix and red wine in the pan and bring up to a simmer. Slice the porcini mushrooms and add them to the pan, together with their soaking liquor (discarding the gritty bit at the bottom of the cup). Mix the cornflour with a little water and add to the pan. Stir well. Simmer for 5 minutes, then reintroduce the beef and simmer for a further 5 minutes before serving with the kale mashed potato.

Cheesy Greens Pasta Bake

526 calories

2
of your SIRT
5 a day

A great family favourite.

Serves 6 • *Ready in 20 minutes*

1 tbsp olive oil

2 shallots, peeled and finely chopped

Large handful (30g) flat-leaf parsley,
stalks finely chopped

400ml milk

30g plain flour

30g butter

30g soft cream cheese

100g mature Cheddar cheese, grated

30g Parmesan cheese, grated

1 × 400g tin butter beans, rinsed and drained

500g fresh fusilli pasta

600ml boiling water

200g baby leaf spinach

40g panko or breadcrumbs

1 Preheat the oven to 240°C (220°C fan/Gas 9).
2 Heat the oil on a low heat in a large ovenproof casserole dish. Add the shallots and parsley stalks and fry gently for 5 minutes until soft.
3 Turn the heat to high and pour in the milk. Add the flour and butter. Now whisk constantly with a balloon whisk until the mixture thickens. Return the heat to low.
4 Add the soft cheese, three-quarters of the Cheddar and about half the Parmesan. Add the butter beans. Continue to heat slowly until all the cheese is melted and incorporated.
5 Turn up the heat to high and add the fresh pasta and boiling water. Return to the boil and cook for 2 minutes. Remove from the heat and stir in the spinach.
6 In a small bowl, combine the breadcrumbs, remaining Cheddar and Parmesan and the parsley leaves. Sprinkle this mix over the cheesy pasta and place immediately in the hot oven. Cook for 4–6 minutes until the topping is golden and bubbling.

Sticky Pork with Apple

314 calories

2
of your SIRT
5 a day

Sweet and sour flavours merge to make this mouthwatering dish.

Serves 2 • *Ready in 20 minutes*

1 tsp olive oil
1 shallot, peeled and very finely sliced
2 × 125g pork steaks
2 apples, cored and cut into eighths
Small handful (10g) flat-leaf parsley, stalks cut finely
1 clove garlic, peeled and crushed
1 tbsp maple syrup
1 tbsp cider vinegar
3 tbsp water
1 tbsp wholegrain mustard

1   Heat the oil in a large frying pan over a medium-high heat. Add the shallot, stir, then add the pork. Fry for 3–4 minutes each side, until browned. Remove the pork from the pan and set aside to rest.

2   Stir in the apple and parsley stalks and turn the heat down to medium-low. Cook for a few minutes until just starting to soften.

3 Stir in the garlic, maple syrup, vinegar and water. Bring to
   a simmer and return the pork to the pan. Spoon some of
   the liquid over the pork and cook gently for 5–10 minutes
   or until the pork is fully cooked. Stir in the mustard and
   parsley leaves before serving.

DESSERTS

If you fancy a little bit of sweetness and decadence after a meal, then try one of these fruity or chocolate delights.

● ● ●

Baked Pomegranate Cheesecake

Blackcurrant Ripple Meringues

Blackcurrant and Raspberry Granita

Chocolate and Blackberry Mini Pavlovas

Extreme Chocolate Mousse

Green Tea Ice Cream

Pomegranate and Blueberry Ice

Individual Chocolate Apple Pies

Blueberry Fool

Very Berry Trifle

Baked Pomegranate Cheesecake

436 calories

½
of your SIRT
5 a day

A very grand recipe. Worthy of a Persian king ... or at least someone who will really appreciate it.

Serves 12 • Ready in 3 hours + 4 hours chilling time

For the crust:

200g pistachios

50g caster sugar

½ tsp ground cardamom

50g butter, melted

For the filling:

500g soft cream cheese

200g caster sugar

30g milk powder

30g plain flour

300ml soured cream

2 eggs, separated

2 tsp vanilla bean paste

3 sheets leaf gelatine

125ml water

For the topping:

250ml pomegranate juice
1 tbsp caster sugar
4 sheets leaf gelatine
150g pomegranate seeds

1 Preheat the oven to 170°C (150°C fan/Gas 3). Line a large loose-bottomed and straight-sided cake tin with a piece of baking parchment on the base.

2 Use a food processor to grind the pistachios, sugar and cardamom together until finely chopped. Pour in the melted butter and combine into a paste. Press into the base of the prepared tin and bake for 8 minutes. Set aside to cool.

3 In a mixer or by hand, cream the cream cheese and caster sugar together. Add the milk powder and flour and mix in thoroughly. Add the soured cream, egg yolks and vanilla. Dissolve the gelatine in the water as per the packet instructions and then add to the cheesecake filling, stirring well.

4 In a clean bowl, beat the egg whites until they are light and fluffy. Carefully fold into the filling mixture.

5 Rub the sides of the cooled cake tin with a little butter, then add the cheesecake filling. Place the tin on a large sheet of foil and crumple the foil around the sides of the tin. Take a roasting tray and fill with 5cm hot water. Place the cheesecake in the tray and bake in the oven (still at 170°C/150°C fan/Gas 3) for approximately 1 hour. Turn the oven off and leave to cool in the oven for another hour (this should stop it from cracking), before leaving to cool completely at room temperature.

6 Heat the pomegranate juice until warm but not bubbling. Stir in the sugar until dissolved. Make up the gelatine according to the packet instructions and add to the pomegranate juice. Allow to cool to room temperature.

7 Pour about a third of the pomegranate topping over the cheesecake and refrigerate for 10 minutes. Repeat with the next third of the juice and refrigerate for another 10 minutes. Finally pour over the final third of the juice, smooth with the back of a spoon and arrange the pomegranate seeds over the top. Cover and refrigerate again for 4 hours.

Blackcurrant Ripple Meringues

229 calories

1
of your SIRT
5 a day

If you can't get hold of blackcurrants, blackberries or raspberries would also work well in this dish.

Serves 6 • Ready in 2 hours

250g blackcurrants, washed and stalks removed
1 heaped tbsp icing sugar
3 large egg whites
100g caster sugar
150ml double cream

☛

1   Preheat the oven to 130°C (110°C fan/Gas ½). Line a baking
    tray with greaseproof paper or a silicone sheet.

2   Place the blackcurrants in a pan with a little cold water.
    Bring to a simmer and cook gently for 10 minutes. Press
    through a sieve, then add the icing sugar while still warm
    and stir to dissolve. Leave to cool.

3   Place the egg whites in a clean bowl and use an electric
    whisk to beat until they form stiff peaks. Continue to beat
    while adding the sugar, a little at a time. Continue to beat
    until the meringues are thick and glossy, then swirl in
    about 2 tablespoons of the fruit purée, but don't stir it in
    completely. Spoon the meringue onto the prepared tray to
    make 12 equal blobs. Bake for 1½ hours, then remove from
    the oven and leave to cool completely.

4   Lightly whip the cream and use to sandwich together the
    meringues in pairs. Serve with the remaining blackcurrant
    sauce drizzled over.

Blackcurrant and Raspberry Granita

172 calories

3
of your SIRT
5 a day

Feel free to substitute the fruit with other black or red berries.

Serves 2 • Ready in 3 hours

150g blackcurrants, washed and stalks removed
150g raspberries
50g icing sugar

1 Blitz the blackcurrants and raspberries in a blender or food processor. Strain through a sieve to remove the skins. Fold the icing sugar into the fruit purée and stir to dissolve. Transfer to an airtight container and freeze for at least 2 hours.

2 Remove from the freezer and rest at room temperature for 10–15 minutes (or use the defrost setting on the microwave for about 30 seconds). Use a fork to crush the mixture into crystals, then serve immediately.

Chocolate and Blackberry Mini Pavlovas

428 calories

2
of your SIRT
5 a day

Perfectly profligate pavlovas.

Serves 8 • Ready in 2 hours

6 large egg whites

200g caster sugar

50g cocoa powder

1 tsp balsamic vinegar

50g good-quality (70%) dark chocolate,
chopped

For the topping:

300ml double cream

100g icing sugar

500g blackberries

30g good-quality (70%) dark chocolate, grated

1 Preheat the oven to 190°C (170°C fan/Gas 5). Line a large
baking tray with baking parchment or a silicone sheet.

2 Place the egg whites in a large clean bowl and whisk
until they form stiff peaks. Beat in the sugar a tablespoon
at a time and continue to whisk until stiff and glossy.

Add the cocoa, balsamic vinegar and chocolate. Gently fold in until combined.

3 Scoop the meringue into eight roughly even portions on the baking tray and flatten the top of each one. Place in the oven and shut the door, then immediately reduce the oven temperature to 160°C (140°C fan/Gas 3) and cook for approximately 45 minutes. When cooked the meringues should be firm and crunchy on the sides and top, but should still be a little squidgy inside. Turn the oven off, open the door a little and leave to cool slowly in the oven for another half an hour.

4 Remove the meringues to individual serving plates. Whisk the cream until thick enough to hold its own shape. Add the icing sugar and whisk again. Pile the cream on top of each meringue and arrange the blackberries on top. Sprinkle over the grated chocolate.

Extreme Chocolate Mousse

375 calories

1½
of your SIRT
5 a day

This dark and decadent chocolate mousse is too good for the kids.

Serves 4 • Ready in 15 minutes + 1–2 hours chilling

170g good-quality (70%) dark chocolate,
broken into small pieces

20g butter

4 large eggs, separated

1 Place a small heatproof bowl over a pan of gently simmering water, making sure the base of the bowl does not touch the water. Place the chocolate and butter in the bowl and warm slowly until nearly melted. Remove from the heat and stir until thick and glossy.

2 Beat the egg yolks lightly and pour a little at a time into the melted chocolate. Stir continuously until the egg yolks are fully incorporated.

3 Put the egg whites in a clean bowl and use an electric whisk to whisk the egg whites until they form stiff peaks. Add a third of the egg whites to the melted chocolate and mix well. Then fold in the rest of the egg whites very gently, trying not to knock the air out of the egg whites. Divide the mousse among four ramekins or small dishes and chill for 1–2 hours before serving.

Green Tea Ice Cream

148 calories

1
of your SIRT
5 a day

This is an authentic green tea recipe from Japan. It is best made in an ice-cream maker, but can also be made by the manual method of removing from the freezer every half an hour (for up to 4 hours) and crushing with a fork.

Serves 6 • Ready in 30 minutes + chilling

600ml semi-skimmed milk

150g caster sugar

Pinch of salt

30g matcha green tea powder

---

1 Place the milk, sugar and salt in a saucepan. Heat on medium until just steaming, then whisk in the green tea powder. Continue to whisk until the mix starts to foam and steam, but remove from the heat before it starts to boil.

2 Cool the mixture in the pan, then transfer to a bowl or jug, cover and refrigerate for 1–2 hours.

3 When fully chilled, transfer to a pre-chilled ice-cream maker and churn for 20–30 minutes, then transfer to an airtight container and freeze. Remove from the freezer 15 minutes before serving.

Pomegranate and Blueberry Ice

55 calories

1½
of your SIRT
5 a day

Refreshing and packed full of SIRTs.

Serves 2 • Ready in 10 minutes

| 1 tsp matcha green tea powder |
| 100g blueberries, fresh or frozen |
| 100ml pomegranate juice |
| 150g ice cubes |

1 Stir the matcha powder into half a cup of hot water until dissolved. Set aside to cool.

2 Use a food processor or blender to purée the blueberries. Add the pomegranate juice, matcha tea and ice cubes and blend until smooth. Serve immediately.

Individual Chocolate Apple Pies

206 calories

1
of your SIRT
5 a day

These fab little chocolate puddings will brighten up any mealtime. Serve hot or cold.

Serves 4 • *Ready in 40 minutes*

4 eating apples, peeled, cored and chopped
into small pieces

Juice of ½ lemon

20g soft light brown sugar

1 tbsp brandy

50ml water

50g icing sugar

1 tbsp cocoa powder

30g ground almonds

1 large egg white

1 Preheat the oven to 160°C (140°C fan/Gas 3).
2 Put the chopped apple in a saucepan with the lemon juice, brown sugar, brandy and water. Bring to the boil, reduce the heat and cook, covered, for 5 minutes. Uncover, turn the heat up and cook for a further 5 minutes until the sauce has thickened. ☞

3 Mix the icing sugar, cocoa and ground almonds together in a bowl.

4 In a clean bowl, whisk the egg white until it forms stiff peaks, then fold into the dry ingredients.

5 Divide the cooked apple into four individual serving dishes or ramekins. Spoon the topping over the apple and give it a gentle shake or tap to level the mixture.

6 Place the ramekins on a baking tray and bake for 20 minutes.

Blueberry Fool

191 calories

1
of your SIRT
5 a day

A lovely easy treat that can be kept in the fridge until you are ready to eat.

Serves 4 • Ready in 10 minutes + 30 minutes chilling

500g blueberries
400g natural yogurt
50ml crème fraîche
Zest of 2 lemons (washed in hot soapy water to remove wax first)
½ tsp ground cinnamon
30g icing sugar

1 Set aside a handful of blueberries for the top of the fools.
2 Place the rest of the blueberries in a food processor or blender and whizz until smooth. If you prefer you can strain the blueberries through a sieve at this stage to remove the skins.
3 Mix the yogurt, crème fraîche, lemon zest, ground cinnamon and icing sugar together thoroughly in a bowl. Fold in the blueberry sauce very gently to make pleasing swirls.
4 Divide the fool into four serving glasses or ramekins and top with the reserved blueberries. Chill for at least 30 minutes before serving.

Very Berry Trifle

315 calories

1
of your SIRT
5 a day

This delicious trifle absolutely thrills my children every time I make it.

Serves 8 • Ready in 20 minutes + 1 hour chilling

250g strawberries, hulled and roughly chopped
250g raspberries
250g blackcurrants, washed and stalks removed
50g caster sugar
100ml water

50ml kirsch or sherry

200g plain sponge cake

200ml double cream

200g custard

1 Put the strawberries, raspberries and blackcurrants in a saucepan, together with the sugar and 100ml water. Bring to the boil and simmer for 10 minutes. Remove from the heat and stir in the kirsch or sherry. Separate the juice from the berries by pouring through a sieve, keeping both.

2 Pour the juice into the bottom of a large glass serving bowl. Cut the sponge into small pieces and push the sponge into the juice at the bottom of the bowl to make a generous layer. Place half the berries on top.

3 Lightly whip the cream and divide into two. Mix half the cream in with the custard and pour over the trifle, then add the rest of the cooked berries. Finally, top with the remaining whipped cream. Cover and refrigerate for at least an hour before serving.

CAKES AND BAKING

One of my favourite things about the SIRT Diet is that you can include some amazing cakes as part of your 'diet'. Following the old adage that everything in moderation is good, these cakes as well as tasting delicious all contain SIRT-rich ingredients, such as cocoa, chocolate, apples and berries. Enjoy!

● ● ●

Chocolate and Lime Truffles

Blackcurrant and Orange Cake

Chocolate Black-Bean Brownies

Cocoa and Grape Cereal Bars

Apple and Blackberry Cake

Kale Savoury Muffins

Chocolate Cupcakes with Matcha Icing

Green Tea and Choc Chip Loaf

Strawberry and Apple Traybake

Double Chocolate and Blackcurrant Muffins

Chocolate and Lime Truffles

64 calories each

3 is
1
of your SIRT
5 a day

These delicious and rich truffles can also be made with rum, kirsch or brandy for a totally different flavour combination.

Makes 20 truffles • Ready in 50 minutes + 30 minutes chilling

100g good-quality (70%) dark chocolate, broken into pieces

50ml double cream

50g unsalted butter, cut into small pieces

Juice and zest of ½ lime (washed in hot soapy
water to remove wax first)

30g cocoa powder

1 Heat a small saucepan of water to near boiling point. Place a bowl on top of the saucepan so it is resting on the rim and near but not touching the boiling water. Add the dark chocolate and double cream to the bowl and warm gently until the chocolate has completely melted into the cream. Remove from the heat.

2 Add the cubed butter and keep stirring until the butter has fully incorporated and the mixture is thick and glossy. Add the lime juice and zest. Whip the mixture using a balloon whisk or similar for 3–5 minutes until it is thick and mousse-like.

3 Cover and refrigerate for at least 30 minutes.

4 Place the cocoa in a shallow bowl. Remove heaped teaspoons of the thickened mixture and roll gently in your hands to make a ball. Roll the ball in the cocoa until it is fully covered. Remove to a plate. Then repeat to make approximately 20 truffles. Keep the truffles in the fridge until needed, but they taste better if rested at room temperature for 10–20 minutes before eating.

Blackcurrant and Orange Cake

261 calories

½
of your SIRT
5 a day

This is an absolutely fabulous cake that contains the lovely SIRTs found in blackcurrants and oranges. It's an easy, hard-to-go-wrong cake and very good if you've got guests to impress. This cake also freezes well.

Serves 12 • Ready in 1 hour

100g butter, at room temperature
150g caster sugar
2 large eggs
200g self-raising flour
¼ tsp ground cinnamon
Tiniest pinch of ground cloves
½ tsp bicarbonate of soda
100g blackcurrants, washed and stalks removed

50g flaked almonds

Zest of 1 orange (washed in hot soapy water to remove wax first)

100ml soured cream

For the glaze:

Juice of 1 orange

50g granulated sugar

1. You will need a medium-sized bundt tin (tube tin) or bake in a normal round tin, giving the cake about 5 minutes extra cooking time. Preheat the oven to 160°C (140°C fan/ Gas 3). Lightly grease the tin.

2. Cream together the butter and caster sugar until light and fluffy. Add the eggs one at a time, beating well after each addition.

3. Add the flour, cinnamon, cloves and bicarbonate of soda and mix well. Fold in the blackcurrants, flaked almonds and orange zest. Finally, fold in the soured cream.

4. Scrape the batter into the prepared tin and level by tapping the pan lightly on the counter. This also releases trapped air bubbles.

5. Bake for 45–50 minutes, until golden brown on top and a skewer inserted in the middle of the cake comes out clean. Leave to cool in the pan for 10–15 minutes and turn out onto a cooling rack.

6. Combine the orange juice and sugar in a small bowl. Use a fork to make multiple holes all over the still warm cake. Spoon and drizzle the glaze all over the top of the cake and then leave to cool completely.

Chocolate Black-Bean Brownies

262 calories

1
of your SIRT
5 a day

With SIRTs in the cocoa, black beans and dark chocolate, there are a lot of SIRTs in these gluten- and wheat-free brownies.

Makes 16 brownies • *Ready in 40 minutes*

2 × 400g tins black beans, rinsed and drained
15ml vanilla bean paste
½ tsp salt
6 large eggs
200g butter, at room temperature
100g dark brown sugar
100g caster sugar
100g cocoa powder
2 tsp baking powder
100g good-quality (70%) dark chocolate chips

1 Preheat the oven to 180°C (160°C fan/Gas 4). Lightly grease a 20cm square cake tin.
2 Place the beans, vanilla bean paste, salt and two eggs in a food processor or blender and blend until smooth.
3 Put the butter, brown sugar and caster sugar in a mixing bowl and beat with a wooden spoon until creamy. Beat in

the remaining eggs one at a time. Add the cocoa powder and baking powder and mix thoroughly. Finally, fold in the bean mixture together with the chocolate chips.

4 Scoop the mixture into the prepared tin, level with the back of the spoon and bake for about 30 minutes. Cool completely in the tin, then tip out onto a chopping board and cut into squares.

Cocoa and Grape Cereal Bars

161 calories

½ of your SIRT 5 a day

These are great for breakfast or as a snack anytime.

Serves 15 • Ready in 50 minutes

400ml tin condensed milk
Few drops of vanilla extract
50g cocoa powder
250g porridge oats
100g red grapes, quartered

1 Preheat the oven to 160°C (140°C fan/Gas 3). Lightly grease a 20cm square cake tin.

2 Heat the condensed milk with the vanilla extract on a low heat in a non-stick pan. Heat until lightly steaming but not bubbling. Meanwhile, mix the cocoa powder to

a smooth paste with a little boiling water. When fully dissolved, add to the condensed milk.

3 Place the oats in a large bowl and stir in the steaming condensed milk. Add the grapes to the bowl, then mix thoroughly. Scoop the mixture into the prepared tin and press down firmly and evenly with the back of a spoon. Bake in the oven for approximately 40 minutes.

4 Remove from the oven and transfer to a chopping board. With a very sharp knife, cut into three in one direction and into five in the other direction, making a total of 15 bars. Transfer to a rack to cool completely. Will keep in an airtight container for up to 6 days.

Apple and Blackberry Cake

249 calories

½
of your SIRT
5 a day

An easy all-in-one cake with SIRT-rich apples and blackberries.

Serves 12 • Ready in 1 hour + cooling time

250g self-raising flour
½ tsp ground cinnamon
90g butter, melted
100g light brown sugar
150ml semi-skimmed milk

2 large eggs, lightly whisked

4 eating apples, peeled, cored and cut into 8 wedges

250g blackberries

For the topping:

50g butter, cut into small cubes

30g light brown sugar

1. Preheat the oven to 190°C (170°C fan/Gas 5). Lightly grease a large (22cm) loose-bottomed cake tin.
2. Sift the flour and cinnamon into a large bowl. Add the butter, sugar, milk and eggs. Mix together well with a wooden spoon. A perfectly smooth texture is not necessary for the texture of this simple cake. Pour into the tin.
3. Arrange the apple wedges over the cake and distribute the blackberries evenly over the top. Dot the cubes of butter over the apple pieces and sprinkle on the sugar. Bake in the oven for approximately 50 minutes, or until a skewer comes out clean. Allow to cool in the tin for at least 15 minutes before removing to a cooling rack. Keeps in an airtight container for up to 3–4 days.

Kale Savoury Muffins

193 calories

1
of your SIRT
5 a day

These are soft, crumbly and delicious. The best thing about muffins is that it's best not to stir too much. A lumpy, lightly folded batter makes the best muffins.

Makes 12 • *Ready in 30 minutes*

40g pine nuts
200g plain flour
40g jumbo oats
2 tsp baking powder
½ tsp bicarbonate of soda
1 tsp salt
Freshly ground black pepper
60g strong Cheddar cheese, grated
100g kale leaves, stalks removed and finely chopped
2 large eggs
250g yogurt
4 tbsp olive oil
100g tomatoes, roughly chopped
20g olives, pitted and roughly chopped

1 Preheat the oven to 200°C (180°C fan/Gas 6) and line a muffin tin with 12 muffin cases. Add the pine nuts to a dry frying pan and heat on high, shaking the pan gently every 30 seconds until the pine nuts are lightly toasted. Leave to cool.

2 In a large bowl, thoroughly mix together the flour, oats, baking powder, bicarbonate of soda, salt, pepper, Cheddar, kale and pine nuts.

3 In another bowl, lightly whisk the eggs with a fork. Add the yogurt, olive oil, tomatoes and olives. Mix well.

4 Pour the egg mix over the flour and fold in until roughly combined. Scoop the mix into the muffin tin and bake for 18–20 minutes until a skewer inserted into the least browned muffin comes out clean. Cool in the tin for 5 minutes, then transfer to a cooling rack to cool completely. Best eaten within 2 days or freeze and defrost as and when you need them.

Chocolate Cupcakes with Matcha Icing

234 calories

1
of your SIRT
5 a day

Simply awesome!

Makes 12 • Ready in 35 minutes + cooling time

150g self-raising flour
200g caster sugar
60g cocoa powder
½ tsp salt
½ tsp fine espresso coffee, decaf if preferred
120ml milk
½ tsp vanilla extract
50ml vegetable oil
1 egg
120ml boiling water

For the icing:

50g butter, at room temperature
50g icing sugar
1 tbsp matcha green tea powder
½ tsp vanilla bean paste
50g soft cream cheese

1 Preheat the oven to 180°C (160°C fan/Gas 4). Line a cupcake tin with 12 paper or silicone cake cases.

2 Place the flour, sugar, cocoa, salt and espresso powder in a large bowl and mix thoroughly.

3 Add the milk, vanilla extract, vegetable oil and egg to the dry ingredients and use an electric mixer to beat until well combined. Carefully pour in the boiling water slowly and beat on a low speed until fully combined. Use a high speed to beat for a further minute to add air to the batter. The batter is much more liquid than a normal cake mix. Have faith, it will taste amazing!

4 Spoon the batter evenly into the cake cases. Each cake case should be no more than three-quarters full. Bake in the oven for 15–18 minutes, until the mixture bounces back when tapped. Remove from the oven and allow to cool completely before icing.

5 To make the icing, cream the butter and icing sugar together until it's pale and smooth. Add the matcha powder and vanilla and stir again. Finally, add the cream cheese and beat until smooth. Pipe or spread over the cakes.

Green Tea and Choc Chip Loaf

313 calories

1
of your SIRT
5 a day

Using matcha powder gives this cake an unusual, delicate flavour.

Serves 8 • Ready in 1 hour

100g butter, at room temperature
120g caster sugar
2 large eggs
½ tsp vanilla extract
50ml milk
150g self-raising flour
1 tbsp matcha green tea powder
100g good-quality (70%) dark chocolate chips

1 Preheat the oven to 180°C (160°C fan/Gas 4). Lightly grease a loaf tin. Cut a long strip of baking parchment the width of the loaf tin. Place the parchment strip so that it covers the base and two ends of the tin, leaving extra at both ends to allow you to pull the cake neatly out of the tin after baking.

2 Cream the butter and sugar together until pale and creamy. Add the eggs one at a time, beating after each. Stir in the vanilla and milk.

3 In a separate bowl, sieve the flour. Stir in the matcha powder and chocolate chips until evenly distributed. Pour in the wet ingredients and fold together until combined.

4 Pour the batter into the prepared loaf tin and bake for approximately 40–45 minutes, or until a skewer comes out clean. Cool in the tin for a short while before picking up by the baking parchment 'handles' and transferring to a cooling rack. This cake keeps well for several days and can be frozen.

Strawberry and Apple Traybake

326 calories

½
of your SIRT
5 a day

Strawberries, apples and blueberries all contain SIRTs.

Makes 12 • Ready in 1 hour + cooling time

200g butter, at room temperature
250g caster sugar
3 large eggs
100ml natural yogurt
250g self-raising flour
2 cooking apples, peeled, cored and sliced
150g strawberries, hulled and halved
50g blueberries

1 Preheat the oven to 190°C (170°C fan/Gas 5). Lightly grease a 20cm × 30cm non-stick cake tin.

2 Cream the butter and sugar together. Add the eggs one at a time, beating well. Stir in the yogurt, then fold in the flour until you have a (still slightly lumpy) batter.

3 Pour half the mixture into the cake tin and smooth out evenly. Arrange one sliced apple over the cake mix and half of the strawberries and blueberries. Top with the remaining batter and repeat with the remaining apple, strawberries and blueberries.

4 Bake for approximately 45 minutes, or until a skewer comes out clean. Cool for 10–20 minutes in the tin, then cut into 12 pieces. The traybake can be served warm or cooled. When cooled, the cake (or individual slices) can be frozen.

Double Chocolate and Blackcurrant Muffins

229 calories

1
of your SIRT
5 a day

Quick and easy to prepare, everyone loves these muffins.

Makes 12 • Ready in 30 minutes

200g plain flour
40g cocoa powder
2 tsp baking powder
½ tsp bicarbonate of soda
100g dark brown sugar
100g good-quality (70%) dark chocolate, cut into chunks
2 large eggs
50g butter, melted
250g yogurt
200g fresh blackcurrants, washed and stalks

1 Preheat the oven to 200°C (180°C fan/Gas 6) and line a muffin tin with 12 muffin cases.
2 In a large bowl, thoroughly mix together the flour, cocoa powder, baking powder, bicarbonate of soda, brown sugar and chocolate chunks.

3 In another bowl, lightly whisk the eggs with a fork. Mix in the melted butter slowly, then stir in the yogurt.

4 Pour the egg mix over the flour and fold in until roughly combined. Carefully fold in the blackcurrants. Scoop the mix into the muffin tin and bake for 18–20 minutes until a skewer comes out clean.

5 Cool in the tin for 5 minutes, then transfer to a cooling rack to cool completely. Best eaten within 2 days or freeze and defrost as and when you need them.

ACKNOWLEDGEMENTS

Thanks to my husband and kids for their totally honest recipe reviews.

AUTHOR BIO

Jacqueline Whitehart is the author of several successful cookbooks and runs a popular healthy-eating blog www.52recipes.co.uk with 100s of fabulous and free healthy recipes. Jacqueline lives in Yorkshire with her husband and three children.

INDEX